FLYING

OVER THE FINISH LINE

Patt and Howard,

One of the principles
of Flying relates to
the value of Support
teams. You are such
important members of
so many support teams –
for each other and
your family.

All the best,

Love,

Sue

Susan L Kane

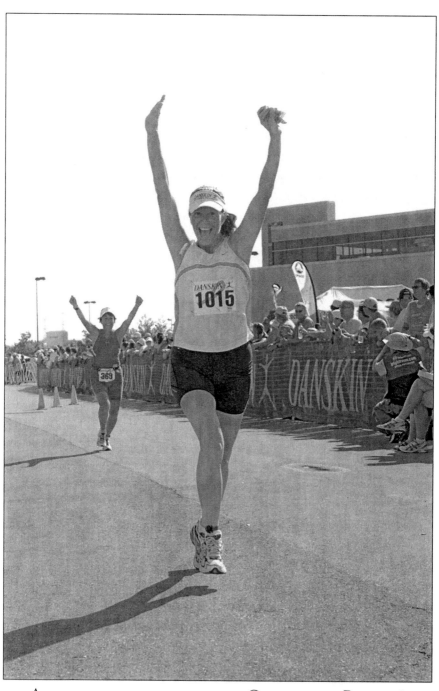

A JUBILANT FINISHER AT THE 2007 CHICAGOLAND DANSKIN!
(PHOTO COURTESY OF BRIGHTROOM.COM)

FLYING OVER THE FINISH LINE

Women Triathletes' Stories of Life

Susan L. Kane

Foreword by

Sally Edwards
National Spokeswoman
Danskin® Women's Triathlon Series

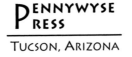

PENNYWYSE PRESS
Tucson, Arizona

Published in the United States of America by:

Pennywyse Press
3710 East Edison Street
Tucson, AZ 85716

"A Prayer for a Friend" by Rhoda-Katie Hannan. Copyright © 1985 by Blue Mountain Arts, Inc. Reprinted by permission. All rights reserved.

"Navigating Life's Transitions" by Mary Ann Bailey, MC. Bailey Coaching. Reprinted by permission.

Library of Congress Cataloging-in-Publication Data

Flying over the finish line : women triathletes' stories of life / [compiled by] Susan L. Kane ; foreword by Sally Edwards.
    p. cm.
  ISBN 978-0-9799341-4-8 (pbk. : alk. paper)
  1. Triathlon. 2. Women athletes—Anecdotes. 3. Women athletes—Biography. I. Kane, Susan L.
  GV1060.73.F589 2008
  796.42'57--dc22
                    2008016168

ISBN 978-0-9799341-4-8

Book Design by Leila Joiner, Imago Press, www.imagobooks.com
Editing by Robin Quinn, Brainstorm Editorial, www.writingandediting.biz

Printed in the United States of America on Acid-Free Paper

For more info, visit www.couragetotri.com.

To Mark,
My forever love.
You are the wind beneath my wings.
I will always be grateful for
your encouragement and support
that frees me to Fly.

"Go confidently into the direction of your dreams!

Live the life you always imagined."

– Thoreau

Contents

DISCLAIMERS

Acknowledgements

My heartfelt gratitude goes out to so many for their contributions and support, which transformed *Flying Over the Finish Line* from a dream to a reality. My special thanks is extended to:

Sally Edwards, my friend and mentor. As the National Spokeswoman for the Danskin Women's Triathlon Series, she has inspired tens of thousands of women to fly over the finish line. Well aware that I would always be a "middle of the packer," she recognized something in me and encouraged me to Fly.

All those who contributed their stories, opening their hearts and lives to others, often based on an email request from a total stranger (me!). Though not all the stories submitted were incorporated into *Flying Over the Finish Line*, I was touched by each and every story I received.

The numerous Team Danskin Training Coaches who encouraged their training team members to share their stories with me, as well as Joy Hermsen, who rallied the coaches to have their team members submit their stories and shared others that she had collected.

The many women associated with the University of Chicago Women's Business Group (UCWBG), including the inspiring women leaders who were keynote speakers at our events, board members, and the members at large. Many of the life lessons I've learned were influenced by the thought leaders who were part of the UCWBG.

My editor, Robin Quinn, who seemingly dropped everything to assist me in getting my book project to the finish line. Her expert recommendations, choice words and cheery disposition were just what I needed to meet the final project deadlines. Thanks also to Syd Mooney of Quinn's Word for Word for her timely proofread at the final stages.

My sister-in-law Keri Stanley, who first introduced me to the Danskin Women's Triathlon Series and challenged me to tri. The many friends who have tri-ed with me over the years: Peggy Olson

(I couldn't ask for a better friend), Jean Spiegelhalter (who always challenged me on our bike rides and was a terrific coaching partner), Karen Seibert (who set the pace on our runs), Christine Cantarino (the busy business executive who amazingly found the time to tri). I hope to find each of you at a start line with me again.

My Mom and Dad, Rosemary and Elliott Satinover. From an early age, with their encouragement, I learned I could do whatever I set my mind to. Special thanks to my Mom for her meticulous proofreading of my (many) early drafts. My father-in-law, Jerry Kane, who has often been at triathlon finish lines to see me fly and has been a constant supporter of my book. I know my mother-in-law Arlene is looking down with pride, knowing I finished the project we talked about over two years ago.

Last, but not least, thanks to my immediate family. To my husband Mark, and children Gregg, Matt and Carly—thanks for understanding as I sat by the computer for hours on end. To Carly, especially, for communicating her admiration for my taking on this project as well as the many triathlons. To Mark, who's been there as I've crossed so many finish lines, for understanding and accepting that I rarely take the easy path and that challenges and goals are a critical component of who I am. For always loving and supporting me—knowing that it's far easier at some times than at others.

P.S. I would be remiss if I didn't acknowledge the Danskin Women's Triathlon Series, which, under the leadership of VP of Sports Marketing and Series Director Maggie Sullivan, provides this amazing venue to women like me and those whose stories are included in *Flying Over the Finish Line*. This event creates a special space for women where they can realize strengths and abilities of their own that they never knew existed until they had the opportunity to fly over the finish line of a Danskin Women's Triathlon.

Foreword

Are You Ready to Take Flight? (Say "Yes!")

by Sally Edwards,
Professional triathlete, best-selling author,
and National Spokeswoman of the
Danskin® Women's Triathlon Series

Like exercise, reading a book is medicine. And this magnificent book, *Flying Over the Finish Line*, is medicine for the heart—that all-important muscle that never misses a beat 24 hours a day, 365 days a year, every year of your life.

In fact, *Flying Over the Finish Line* is medicine for both the heart *and* the soul. Here's a chance for you to reach into women's lives, their challenges, their triumphs, and their motivation in a way that is personal and private, yet also universal in its message. This book has been sculpted by author Susan Kane in such a way that she doesn't get between you and the women athletes. Within these pages, she provides a fresh look at contemporary American women. Often today's woman travels a long and winding road before finding the real person inside who has been waiting for her all along.

Susan Kane is one of those women who has traveled that long and winding road. Already a businesswoman, mother and wife, Susan added "athlete" and later "author" to her list. After traveling down her own path of discovery, while overcoming medical challenges, struggles with the great balancing act of family, career and taking care of herself, after wrestling with her own fears and anxieties, she gathered the stories of over 50 women, weaving them into a cohesive whole with intrigue that keeps you reading—from beginning to end.

As you read, you'll understand why Susan is so passionate and committed to sharing the stories of the many women who chose the swim-bike-run triathlon to transition their lives from wherever they were to the finish line. You'll come to understand that there is one core message for every woman who is part of this tale. This is that you can realize your dream of flying across the finish line—you can turn dreams into reality. You'll hear this theme in every triathlete's story, and it is exciting enough to give you chills. In reading these pages, you'll share in feeling what everyday women experience traveling from the starting line to the finish line—from regular gal to triathlete finisher. It is a feeling of takeoff, of gaining elevation, of soaring, and then of being emancipated.

Susan shares this journey in the voices of each of the women who volunteered to come forward and boldly share her life with you—including Susan's own transition and transformation as a woman who, like the others in *Flying Over the Finish Line*, learns the personal power and freedom that comes from taking flight.

If there's a secret buried in the pages of *Flying Over the Finish Line*, it is this: if you haven't read this book, you are at a disadvantage to those who have enjoyed every single real story that Susan has included. Of all of the reasons why so many miss the discovery that exercise is medicine, that it can be a cure for so many ills, the real reason often is a lack of motivation to try one more time to get fit. Read on. You're sure to gain the motivation to give exercise one more try by turning these pages.

Also, if you've experienced what so many other women have on the road to their goal—failure or disappointment after losing to the ever-present obstacles of life, the need for courage, or the inability to fully identity with your vision of that "new you" of the future—then *Flying Over the Finish Line* may be your best medicine, your cure.

Are you ready to read how so many women do it? Are you ready to find that wonderful woman inside who is waiting for you? Are you ready to meet others who have accomplished what they thought was never possible? Are you ready to make the dream of embracing your inner athlete come true? Do you long to transform other life goals into reality? Are you ready to fly over the finish line? I believe that you're more than ready, and to fuel your flight, I wholeheartedly recommend that you read this book.

Sally Edwards
May 12, 2008
Sacramento, California

P.S. Susan Kane became my friend and inspiration when she reached deep into her pocket to find a one-dollar bill. She invested it into the winning raffle ticket for my favorite charity, Team Survivor USA (www.teamsurvivor.org), an organization for women who have survived cancer and use exercise as one of their treatments to recovery. As the winner of the raffle, she did one workout with me—a bike ride to the top of a mountain—and we became lifelong friends. I respect her enormously, and after you read what follows, you will become as big a fan as I am!

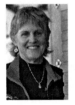 Sally Edwards, MA, MBA, is one of America's leading experts in business, exercise science, and lifestyle living. She is the innovator behind the Heart Zones Training proprietary and branded training system. Since 1990, she has served as the National Spokeswoman for the Danskin® Women's Triathlon Series, one of the crown jewels of the sport of triathlon. She has completed over 120 Danskin® Triathlons during the past 19 years, volunteering to be the "final finisher" in each so that no other woman has to face being last.

Sally is a best-selling author with more than 20 books and 500 articles on health and fitness. Her books include the popular titles, *Heart Rate Monitor GUIDEBOOK* and *The Complete Book of Triathlons*. This professional triathlete is a 16-time Ironman finisher, a member of the Triathlon Hall of Fame, and past winner of the Western States 100 Mile Endurance Run.

She is a sought-after professional speaker, delivering dozens of presentations each year. Today, Sally uses her passion for getting America fit to lead The Sally Edwards Company, a media company dedicated to uncommonly vibrant lifestyles, and Heart Zones USA, an international training, education, and coaching company. Sally Edwards is an example of what she teaches—living an active healthy lifestyle—which, in her case, takes place in Sacramento, California.

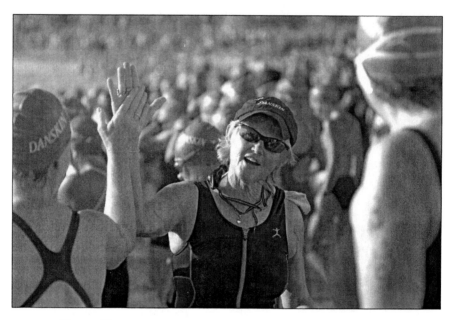

SALLY EDWARDS HIGH-FIVES BEFORE THE SWIM START.
(PHOTO COURTESY OF BRIGHTROOM.COM)

Introduction

The Start of My Amazing Journey

One night over a family dinner, my 10-years-younger, athletic sister-in-law, Keri Stanley, told me about the Danskin Women's triathlon she planned to do. Keri urged me to join her. At first, I laughed. *Me?* I was 42 years old. Though I had worked out regularly as an adult to avoid the Battle of the Bulge, I was not involved in athletics growing up—never joined a sports team or had a coach. Over the next couple of days, I mulled over the idea. With less than three months to train, knowing nothing about the sport of triathlon, I decided to accept the challenge—for reasons I will later describe.

Without a whole lot of guidance, I started training in swimming, biking and running. I had a fairly new mountain bike (with a little rack on the back) that I used for an occasional three-mile ride to my office. It would serve the purpose just fine. I used to run now and then, so that was the easy part. Later in the book, you'll hear about how I developed my swim skills.

The night before the triathlon, after picking up my race number during the day, I was in a panic. *What was I thinking? I was going to do what? I had never set an athletic goal in my life—why did I think I could do this?*

Despite my fear and self-doubt, I made it to the start line the next morning—probably because I had recruited a couple of friends and I couldn't let these budding triathletes down. Two hours and two minutes after the start of my wave (my group of participants), I flew across the finish line of my first Danskin triathlon. It took me exactly twice as long as the professional athlete who won the race that year, but did I care? Actually, it was one of the most empowering moments of my life! I had set a goal totally out of my comfort zone. I had worked hard to prepare. I did something for the first time—a triathlon, no less. I did it! I sobbed uncontrollable tears of joy. I was not the same woman who had started the race.

Since then, there's been no looking back. Triathlons have become an established part of what I do, an important part of who I am. As of this writing, I have completed nine Danskin triathlons at different locations throughout the US, and two international-distance triathlons. And I'm not done yet!

My Life's Twists and Turns

I am a contemporary woman who shares the same challenge that so many other women face each day. That is, trying to create a life that fulfills many competing needs—in my case, keeping a long-standing marriage alive, raising three children, and continuing a career in a way that makes sense for me in light of all my family requirements. I also try to take care of myself and make time for family, friends, fun and laughter.

At times in my past, I've led a pretty stressed-out life, trying to do it all (and do it to perfection, no less!). Admittedly, much of that pressure has been self-imposed. I was never especially good at "settling." I wanted it *all*. It was my choice to continue my career rather than stay home full-time with my three children. It was important to me that my home was nicely decorated and "company clean." I wouldn't allow "letting myself go" appearance-wise. I even chose to go back to grad school at the University of Chicago GSB, entering one of the most challenging MBA programs in the country and then having my third child halfway through the required classes for the degree.

All of these demands on my life ultimately took their toll on my health. At the age of 34, when I appeared to have it all—a hardworking, loving husband, three healthy and smart kids, an impressive job, a beautiful new home—I was afflicted with a rare autoimmune disease that affected my kidneys. It was a disease that my nephrologist (kidney specialist) told me had no known cause. According to traditional medicine, there was nothing I could do to prevent a recurrence. Although stress might have been a contributing factor, it was likely just one of the lemons that had lined up on the slot machine of my life to cause the disease. The other lemons were unknown. The disease would just need to be treated (with high dosages of steroids) and I could pray that it would go away, never to return.

The six or seven months of steroid treatments were extremely tough. In the midst of my journey back to health, the venture-funded software company I was working for began a quick spiral downward. This soon meant that I was out of a job a year after we had moved into our new home, complete with the accompanying big mortgage payments. Needless to say, it was an extremely challenging time. One of the lessons I learned from that taxing period was to never take my health for granted: *how difficult life was without my health!*

Eventually, I regained my health and found a new job. Finding the right "balance" between my family, health and career continued to be a struggle.

In subsequent years, I had *three* recurrences of my kidney disease. Perhaps surprisingly to some of you, I ended up doing my first "Danskin" in 2000, at the tail end of treatment for my third bout. That was when Keri challenged me to join her in the Danskin triathlon.

At the time, I hated being labeled as a "sickly" person. But how could I be sickly if I became a triathlete? By focusing on keeping my health a top priority, I knew I'd become stronger. Accepting the Danskin challenge was a way to prove to myself and others that I was not willing to be a victim.

Inspired to Tell Our Stories

At my sixth Danskin triathlon, I made it a point to talk with other women to find out why they were there. I believed there had to be so much more to the triathlon's appeal than simply women wanting to be in shape.

For instance, before the start of the early morning swim, I talked to the woman next to me. She told me that her son was stationed in Iraq. Since he had to stay physically fit as part of his job, she decided to focus on her physical fitness by training for the Danskin, and even dedicated the race to her son. That woman touched my heart and was a major source of inspiration for this book! Another woman told me she had weighed 250 pounds the year before, when she began training for a marathon. During the course of that marathon training, she began to lose the weight. The Danskin was the next phase in creating a better life for herself.

In the afternoon, as I recovered from the morning's triathlon experiences, a lightening bolt went off in my head: I needed to collect women's stories to share in an inspirational book! I realized that every woman who does a triathlon has a story that is far beyond the physical fitness aspect of the race. I decided that by gathering and sharing those stories, I could touch other hearts and inspire women to learn from what was said. Soon thereafter, I ran the idea by my friend and mentor, Sally Edwards, the National Spokeswoman for the Danskin Women's Triathlon Series. She has supported me ever since in creating this collection of stories.

After each Danskin, Sally receives letters and emails from Danskin triathletes, sharing the experiences of empowerment that come from flying across the finish line. During the triathlons, she talks with many women who affirm the value of "doing the Danskin." Many of the stories included in this book were initially sent to Sally in appreciation for the inspiration she has provided to so many Danskin women.

A Challenge Ignites a Passion

Writing this book, which has had many stops and starts, was a way of creating a new challenge for myself. I had reached the point where I knew I could complete whatever triathlon I signed up for. I was also realistic about my natural athletic skills (or lack thereof, as my husband might lovingly point out). Being a top finisher in my age group was not likely for me. A new challenge related to my passion for triathlon found voice through this book.

I also integrated my passion for triathlon into my life by becoming a head coach for Team Danskin WTS Training for the Chicago Northwest Suburbs (after a whole lot of arm-twisting by Sally). 2007 was my first year. Through this eight-week program, the "official training program of the DWTS," I was able to share what I'd learned in my previous years of triathlon. It provided the opportunity to work with the many Workout Leaders (WOLs) who volunteer to support the training team. I found new inspiration from these women who willingly shared their knowledge and were only rewarded with the satisfaction of helping someone else. I found further inspiration, too, in the stories of my team members, each of whom had her own reason for tri-ing.

My first training team included 11 delightfully diverse and motivated women. They ranged in age from 29 to 54 (or thereabout, but who's counting?). The team included one stay-at-home mom with young children, doing something for herself. Some teammates seemed to have a personal challenge or obstacle during the entire course of the training. One amazing woman joined the team because she was determined to return to her second triathlon to improve her performance from her first, "when I didn't have a clue what I was doing." This was despite the fact that she had recently been involved in a serious car accident. She was still on crutches for our first team meeting! (Yes, I did make sure she had her doctor's approval before she started training.) Another normally outgoing, vivacious team member dealt with her son's drug overdose just days before the Danskin. She made it to the start line to take care of herself.

I could go on. Each of my team members had a story about why they decided to do the Danskin and the obstacles they had to overcome to make it to the start line. You'll read some of their stories later in this book. My original inspiration to write this book—believing that every woman who decides to do the Danskin has a reason be-yond the physical accomplishment—was affirmed by the experiences of each of the members on my training team.

Ultimately, despite the scheduling conflicts and demands on their time, every one of my training team members made it to the start line of the Chicagoland Danskin and, having been properly trained (heart rate monitors and all), flew across the finish line. It was a great experi-ence for each one of them. It was an even greater experience for me.

In giving to my team members, I received so much in return. I had the opportunity to share what I'd learned from my previous triathlons, including info on heart rate monitors, sports nutrition and training plans. Coaching the team was also an outlet for me to share a message of empowerment with other women—we can do whatever we set our minds on doing. My experience as a coach helped me find myself, too. It provided the opportunity to find moments of "flow"—times when I became so engrossed in what I was doing that time passed without my awareness. As a trainer, I was able to use my skills and knowledge in a new and challenging way.

For me, the challenge of my first triathlon evolved into a long-held passion for the sport. Now I have multiple outlets for my enthu-siasm for triathlon—as a competitor (I use that term loosely), writer and coach.

Other Women's Journeys

There are stories from more than 50 women in the pages of my book. Women of all ages, backgrounds, careers and experiences. Their sto-ries inspired me. Some made me laugh. Others brought tears to my eyes. Themes surfaced and repeated in many of the stories. I hope their stories will touch your heart as they have touched mine.

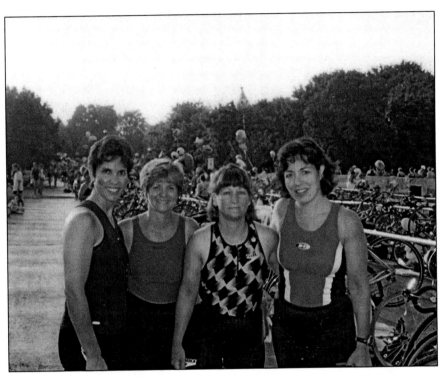

FRIENDS JEAN SPIEGELHALTER, PEGGY OLSON, KAREN SEIBERT, AND SUSAN KANE (LEFT TO RIGHT) SHARE A PEACEFUL MOMENT BEFORE THE START OF THEIR SECOND DANSKIN TRIATHLON.

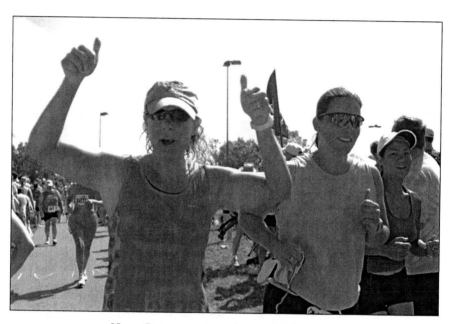

KERI STANLEY AND LAURIE STANLEY
FINISH THE 2007 CHICAGOLAND DANSKIN.

CHAPTER 1

"Flying" 101

Since you've picked up this book, it may be that you're looking for encouragement to complete a triathlon. Perhaps you're considering flying over the finish line yourself because you need a new challenge or want to get into better shape. You've investigated options and might even have specifically discovered the Danskin® Women's Triathlon Series (also referred to as "DWTS," "the Danskin," or "Danskin WTS").

Or maybe you have a friend or family member who's done a triathlon and wants you to join them. Because of your skepticism, the triathlete gave you this book to convince you that you really can do it.

Or perhaps you've already completed your first triathlon or a 5k or another physical challenge you set for yourself. You'd like to do more but from time to time the voice of self-doubt creeps in. *Do I really have the time to train again? To train harder and farther? I've got so many other things to do…* You, too, think a dash of inspiration and encouragement would help.

Still, it's possible that you're reading this book even though setting an athletic goal isn't on your radar screen. Instead, you're looking for inspiration from women who have the mindset to accomplish a triathlon. That's okay, too. If you're looking to be inspired to stretch beyond your current comfort zone, you're in the right place.

You'll learn some specifics about triathlons in this chapter, in case that's your goal. (If not, feel free to jump ahead to the next chapter after reading this paragraph. The women's stories begin in Chapter 2.) I'd bet that you probably already know that triathlons usually include a combination of swimming, biking and running. What you may not realize is that triathlons serve as a great metaphor for life. Lessons women learn from triathlons can be applied to all aspects of our daily lives. As you read the stories throughout the book, you'll be amazed how completing a triathlon helps bring the women to a new level. Tapping their wisdom can help you reach new levels in your life, too, whatever goal is currently calling to you.

An Introduction to Triathlons

If you're new to the sport of triathlon, here are the basics. Triathlons involve three different sports combined into one event. As I've mentioned above, most traditional triathlons consist of a swim, bike, and run.

There are "sprint" triathlons, which are perfect for beginners. Though the actual distances may vary, the most common sprint-distance triathlon will consist of a 1/2-mile swim, a 12-mile bike ride, followed by a 5k (3.1-mile) run. The "international" or "Olympic" distance triathlon approximately doubles those distances with a .9-mile swim, 24.6-mile bike ride and 10k (6.2-mile) run. International distance triathlons are a good goal to move up to once you're comfortable with sprint distance races.

The "granddaddy" of them all—the ultimate triathlon—is the Ironman World Championship. This includes a 2.4-mile ocean swim and a 112-mile bike ride, which are followed by a marathon—a 26.2-mile run! For most of us mere mortals, an Ironman race is something to watch with admiration—but without the slightest expectation of participating. The Ironman concept originated in 1978 and had 15 male participants.[1] Today, participation in the Championship event is limited to 1,700 people, primarily those who have had qualifying times in another of the approximately 20 Ironman races held throughout the world. The Ironman World Championship takes place in Kona on the Big Island of Hawaii. So you'll hear references to "the road to Kona."

There are variations to any of these distances, depending upon the race venue and objectives. There are also other multi-sport variations. An "aquathon," sometimes referred to as an "aquathlon," is a two-stage race with a swim followed by a run. An "aquabike" consists of swimming and biking. Depending on the event, an aquabike event could be as long as the Ironman distances—a 2.4-mile swim followed by a 112-mile bike, without the 26.2-mile run. "Duathlons," which include only two sports, are often structured as run-bike-run.

The appeal of triathlons is that they are challenging and FUN! The challenge comes from training for three *different* sports, with the objective of becoming *proficient* in each. Believe it or not, there is an appeal in that. It's easier on your body than all the pounding involved in training for an endurance running race, for example. As for fun, how can you beat the enjoyment you had as a kid when biking around your hometown—*what freedom!* What a great way to cover distances quickly, as if flying through the air. And swimming, though a challenge for many, brings freedom in the water. Believe it or not, there are many triathletes for whom the swim is the best/easiest part of the triathlon. (I'm not one of them!)

Swim, bike, run. What a fantastic combination! If you're training with a team or friends and family, you can have a great time together. And I've always found the people involved with triathlons—especially the women (we'll get to that)—are really wonderful people to be around.

In case you're wondering who does triathlons—because you're thinking it probably isn't people like you!—here's some information you need to know. Triathlon is the fastest growing sport in the world, according to USA Triathlon ("USAT"), which serves as the national governing body for triathlon, duathlon, aquathon, and winter triathlon in the United States. From 2002 to 2007, the total number of members in USAT nearly doubled from 53,000 to 103,000. In 2002, 16,000 members, 30% of the total, were women. By 2007, nearly 37,000 participants were women—which represent 36% of the total membership. As you can see, women's participation is growing at a faster rate than men's![2,3]

As far as age goes, triathlons are not just for the young. In fact, the majority of female members in USAT are between the ages of 30 and 49. For 2007, there were over 3,000 members 50 and older—including three women in the 80+ age category! (I want to meet those three ladies someday for a real dose of inspiration.)[4]

Other characteristics of triathletes are that they tend to be extremely focused and driven to succeed. The vast majority hold at least 4-year degrees and are employed in professional or managerial positions.[5] But there's no "one size fits all"—especially when you consider the triathletes who participate in the Danskin Women's Triathlon Series.

Increased diversity of triathletes is definitely wanted and needed. People of color currently compose less than one percent of triathletes.[6] Minority participation is encouraged, especially through Team Dream, a Chicago-area based triathlon training team for women of color. Under the leadership of dynamic Derrick Q. Milligan, Team Dream has grown to over 200 members who participate in the Danskin and other triathlons and athletic events.

Hopefully, your stereotypes of triathletes are dissolving and you, too, want to become one—that is, if you haven't already!

What's "the Danskin"?

Most of my own triathlon experiences—certainly all of my *best* triathlon experiences—have come from completing sprint-distance triathlons in the Danskin Women's Triathlon Series. Since 1990, Danskin Inc., the women's activewear company, has been sponsoring a triathlon series exclusively for women.

In its initial year, the Danskin Women's Triathlon Series included three locations and 1,100 athletes. Since its inception, nearly 200,000 women have crossed the finish line of a Danskin triathlon after swimming a half mile, biking 12, and then running a 5k. Today, over

22,000 women of all shapes and sizes from all walks of life complete the Danskin annually in its eight locations across the US. Participant profiles range from women 14 to 77 years of age and from 90 pounds to 375 pounds. It's the longest running multi-sport series in the world.[7]

The Danskin Women's Triathlon Series is directed by Maggie Sullivan, Danskin VP of Sports Marketing. Providing a safe and memorable experience to each and every Danskin triathlete is paramount to Maggie. Though coordinating the Danskin Series is her job, there's no doubt that Maggie pours her heart into it.

According to Maggie, approximately half of each year's participants are first-timers. That means the other half are returning. Why do women try the Danskin? Because of the safe, supportive environment it provides. Everyone who is there wants every woman to succeed. Why do women return to the Danskin? Because the experience transcends the sport itself.

The phenomenal and enduring growth of "the Danskin" is likely for a reason expressed by many women who complete it—that the event is about so much more than meeting an athletic goal. Many of the women who "do the Danskin" have never considered themselves "athletes" prior to committing to doing the race. But they chose to take it on as a way to create a better life and to learn something about themselves in the process.

The stories of the Danskin participants and other female triathletes provide great inspiration and insight into life. By sharing the stories in this book, I hope to inspire you to look at your own life and examine changes you might make to assure that you're living your best life. This may include doing a triathlon, but it may not.

Reasons to Tri

Let's take a closer look at why you might want to do a triathlon. The most obvious answer would be to get physically fit or improve your current level of fitness. More on that later. Another reason might be to lose some weight. While a triathlon can help with that, exercise alone is not enough. You need to be realistic. To lose weight, proper nutrition is key. You have to combine healthy eating with exercise. You can't just go out and ride your bike for an hour to justify a big burger and large serving of fries. But if you're working out on a regular basis, you'll find new motivation to eat healthily. Slowly and steadily, you'll see real progress.

Another reason to do a triathlon is that you need a goal. Perhaps your life has been on autopilot for a while. You need something new and exciting to do. Committing to your first triathlon will help you stick to your exercise program. In fact, no longer will you be merely exercising or working out. When you're doing those things with a goal in mind, you are TRAINING. And you're much more likely to stick to your TRAINING when you have a specific goal in mind.

Another benefit that comes from completing a triathlon is the sense of accomplishment that comes from completing a stretch goal. How empowering it feels to "do the thing that you think you cannot do," using the famous words of Eleanor Roosevelt. It's amazing to accomplish the seemingly impossible. There will be spillover results into all other aspects of your life.

Benefits of Physical Fitness

Throughout this book, I will emphasize many other benefits of preparing for an athletic event like a triathlon besides becoming physically fit. Still, there's no denying that improved fitness is one of the great payoffs. And as will be reinforced by the varied stories of this book, the positive impacts on your body from becoming physically fit are many. They include:

- **Reducing health risks.** Regular exercise is crucial to reducing blood pressure, cholesterol levels and triglycerides—all markers of heart disease. It can also reduce or eliminate risks associated with diabetes and certain cancers. Those who undergo surgery recover quicker if they are otherwise healthy prior to the surgery. Exercise improves the immune system and increases stress tolerance.

- **Strengthening bones.** Weight-bearing exercises strengthen bones and reduce the risk of osteoporosis. A good triathlon training program will incorporate some work with weights.

- **Improving flexibility.** An exercise program should include stretching to maintain and improve muscle and joint flexibility. Proper stretching before and after running and biking is another important component of a good triathlon training program.

- **Improving sleep.** It's easier to fall asleep and stay slumbering with regular exercise, which renews energy.

- **Controlling aging.** Physical activity and fitness are the most important factors in successfully controlling aging. Once we reach our 40s or 50s, our bodies start to decline unless they receive signals to the contrary. The best way to override the "decline message" is daily exercise, which is a signal for growth. *I'm too old* is not a reason to stay away from triathlon.

When training for a triathlon, we start to feel better about ourselves as we feel physically stronger and healthier. We reach new levels of energy and confidence. How great is that?

Let's Talk about Emotional Fitness

Another benefit of physical activity is that there is a direct relationship between physical fitness and emotional fitness. The neural circuitry for the mind and body (thus the body, thoughts, and emotions) are entwined and interconnected.[8]

Emotional fitness reduces feelings of stress and fatigue and promotes happiness and energy. Physical activity promotes emotional fitness with chemicals called endorphins, which directly impact the brain. The release of endorphins and creation of serotonin in the body bring a sense of optimism and happiness. Exercise has been shown to decrease depression and can be as effective as certain mood-enhancing drugs that are currently prescribed with increasing frequency in our lives. Not that there isn't a place for antidepressant medications, but if you can get a solution that is 100% natural, as may be the case with exercise, why not go for it?

Risk-Taking: Good or Bad?

You understand that exercise and physical fitness can impact your overall attitude in a positive way. You see that having a training program would help you stick to your intended exercise goals. But perhaps you're still not convinced that you should complete a triathlon—because you'd have to move out of your comfort zone. *My life is okay just as it is, right now*, you think.

Well, challenges are a good thing. There's the adage that if you're not moving forward, you're moving backward. You need to move out of your comfort zone now and then. Your brain wants to learn new things. It needs to be challenged. You really can do it! Stretch yourself. Take a risk. Training for a triathlon will take you out of your comfort zone but it isn't an unreasonable or unhealthy risk. You won't regret it.

But What If I Fail?

Perhaps what's holding you back from making the commitment to complete your first triathlon is the fear that you will fail. What if you put yourself out there, commit to participating in a triathlon, and then don't accomplish your goal? What if you FAIL???

First of all, the likelihood of failing—of not finishing a sprint distance triathlon—is small. Once you've set the goal, you will create a plan to achieve it. As long as you follow the plan, the chance of not being successful is pretty minimal. You really CAN do this!

Let's go to the worst-case scenario for a minute. What happens if you *don't* cross the finish line of your first triathlon (or tenth triathlon, for that matter)? That *could* happen for any number of reasons that are totally outside of your control. For example, you get a flat tire while biking or have some other equipment problem that can't be fixed. Or the temperature and humidity on the day of your event is so unbearably hot you just can't finish the race without threat to your health. (As I write this, it is only months after the Chicago Marathon in October 2007 where 9,000 of the 45,000 who registered [and probably trained a great deal] didn't even show up for the race because of exceptional heat. Eleven thousand people crossed the start line but didn't finish because of extreme weather conditions.[9])

It's important to keep in mind that the problems described at the Chicago Marathon occurred for the first time in its 30-year history! If you don't finish your triathlon for whatever reason, you *will* be disappointed. Protecting your safety is certainly not failure. Not achieving your goal is not the end of your life. There will be other events and opportunities. What's important is to figure out what you've learned from your experience to make you better prepared and smarter for your next event. There *will* be a next event.

Another consideration is how you define success and failure. At the Danskin triathlons, I've worked my way up to being a "middle-of-the-packer" athlete. I've also completed two international-distance triathlons to date. I'm usually about the last one in my age group (and the race overall) to finish this distance triathlon. (In the smaller local triathlons, there aren't exactly a whole lot of women in my age group participating.) Now, I could look at that as failure—finishing last or pretty close to it. However, I prefer to applaud myself for being there at all. I'm a winner for just showing up while most other women my age—and younger—are still at home sleeping when I'm waiting at the start line. It's all in how you define your success. The only true failure would be a situation where you don't learn from your experience about doing it better next time. So forget about failing. Minimize your risks and start living!

Minimizing the Risk?

There's plenty you can do to minimize the risk and increase your chances of having a successful experience with triathlon. One way is to enlist the support of your friends and family. If you have friends and family to train with, you're more likely to stick to your training plan. And if you stick to your plan, you can succeed. Also, as we discussed earlier, training with friends and family is more fun.

You can also participate in a formal training program. For the Danskin Women's Triathlon Series, for example, there are a variety of formal training programs to support the triathletes in getting ready for the starting line. That might include participating in a training team such as Heart Zones Team Danskin WTS Training. This comprehensive 8-week program is led by an experienced coach. There are two workouts each week as a team, as well as others you do on your own. Other programs include online coaching via email and one-on-one coaching in person or online. And for most other triathlon events, you can find formal training programs and area triathlon clubs that offer skills clinics and other help to prepare for your goal. A nice bonus is that you're bound to make some new friends in most formal training programs, and these friends can provide further support if it's lacking in your current circle.

Another strategy to ensure success is to set realistic goals. Deciding to train for an Ironman triathlon in the upcoming summer after reading this book probably isn't too realistic—that is, if you're a reader who has never done a triathlon at all. As you'll learn from some of the stories in the later chapters of the book, it may take years of training to work yourself up to doing an Ironman distance triathlon. On the other hand, deciding you're going to do your first sprint-distance tri-athlon during the next two or three months sounds like a great idea.

Danskin's Spokeswoman, Sally Edwards

In writing about triathlons and inspiration, I must mention Sally Edwards. For any woman who's been a part of the Danskin Women's Triathlon Series, it's pretty hard not to have been affected by Sally Edwards' infectious enthusiasm and inspiration. As the National Spokeswoman of the Danskin WTS, Sally leads "store talks" in ad-vance of the regional triathlons to encourage potential first-timers and others that they *can* complete a triathlon. At the Expo the day before each race, Sally once again provides another dose of encour-agement that the hard part—getting to the start line—is over and that you *will* finish the next day. The day of the triathlon, Sally is in the water, offering encouragement as one wave of women after an-other gets in to begin their swim.

Another tradition at the Danskin Triathlons is that Sally is al-ways the final finisher of each race so no one else ever has to worry about being last. Sally accompanies the next-to-last swimmer out of the water and then spends some time at the runners' finish line, con-gratulating women as they fly across. As the race day gets closer to its end, Sally moves out onto the course, accompanying those who are still running toward the finish line, urging them on. Sally is the last woman to cross the finish line.

Sally is a 16-time Ironman Triathlon finisher, including being a former Master's world-record holder (for competitive women 40-49). Instrumental in developing the sport of the triathlon, she is a member of the Triathlon Hall of Fame. Sally is a prolific author of more than 20 titles, and many triathletes have prepared using her books, *The Complete Book of Triathlons* and *Triathlons for Women*. She founded Heart Zones USA, a training and education company which created the original heart-rate training program. Today, she continues to pur-sue her passion to get America fit with The Sally Edwards Company.

There's so much to admire about Sally Edwards. I certainly want to express my appreciation for Sally's support and her willingness to share many wonderful stories of the Danskin women with us.

What Reading This Book *Will* and *Will Not* Do for You

Soon you'll be moving on to the next chapters of *Flying*, where you'll find amazing and inspirational stories of women triathletes. But before then, I want to clarify what this book *is* and what it *is not*.

The book is NOT a "how to" triathlon book. It will not improve any of your triathlon specific skills (unless they're on the "mental side" of the sport, which shouldn't be discounted). There are many good books out there which will help you become a triathlete, or a better triathlete if you've already participated in such an event. I, personally, am partial to Sally Edwards' *Triathlons for Women*. When I prepared for my first few triathlons, there were no training teams to join. Sally's books got me through. Today, there are training teams and triathlon clubs to join, clinics to attend, magazines to read, and websites to peruse.

What this book WILL do for you is to provide a healthy dose of inspiration. You'll read stories from women from all walks of life, who've faced a variety of challenges, yet for one reason or another decided to do a triathlon. You'll feel powerful connections to the women who have shared their stories. You'll ignite a spark of recognition as you see yourself in one or more of the stories. Or you'll read a story that helps you put your own life into perspective. *My challenges are nothing compared to so-and-so's story. If she can do it, so can I.* You'll find a dose of "chicken soup" for the (aspiring) triathlete and so much more.

And what if you're reading this book without any thought of doing a triathlon or other athletic event? Well, you can still definitely benefit from the stories and their accompanying lessons. Many of the experiences presented in the book are universal in their reach. Women have learned lessons from doing the triathlon that apply to their lives much more generally. For instance, over and over again, you'll read, "I learned that if I can do this triathlon, I can do anything I set my mind to doing." In reading the stories of this book, you can learn that you, too, can set your mind to whatever you want—with or without doing a triathlon. So read on and be inspired!

What Is Flying?

If you're new to triathlon, you may be wondering why this book is titled *Flying Over the Finish Line*. After all, aren't we talking about swimming, biking, and running? You don't remember any flying being involved. Perhaps you're finding yourself thinking, *Maybe someone who is young and fast might feel like they're flying, but I'm not too young... will never be fast...*

Flying is a state of mind. If you've completed your first triathlon already, you understand. Flying describes the sense of empowerment that comes from crossing over that finish line, doing something you originally thought was totally out of the realm of possibility. As one Danskin triathlete, Ruth Kaminski, so aptly described, "...it was the soaring and dancing of my spirit rather than the fleetness of my feet."

If one of your self-limiting beliefs is that you are not an "athlete," this book will challenge your thinking. You will hear stories from so many women who, before taking on the Danskin or another triathlon, didn't consider themselves athletes. Regardless of your age, weight, current state of fitness, or whether you were involved in sports when you were growing up, your "inner athlete" resides in you—and is waiting to be freed if physical fitness has been on the back burner for too long. Your inner athlete is someone who wants to make fitness part of each and every day. She longs to fly over a finish line of some kind, and it doesn't have to be a triathlon if you're inspired to engage in physical activity of some other type.

If you're preparing for an athletic event, you'll find strength from the women's experiences in creating and following through on a plan for success. You'll learn ways to create and maintain the motivation to attain your goal, even though unforeseen obstacles may get in the way. You'll be reminded to get rid of the self-limiting voices that prevent you from moving forward. Be assured that the advice shared in this book is based on the real world in which today's busy women live.

In reading these wonderful stories, I hope that you, too, will be encouraged and inspired to take flight. Move outside your comfort zone. Stretch yourself. Do the thing you think you cannot do. Experience the empowerment that comes from flying over the finish line, whatever that means to you.

Because, once you do, you'll realize that you can achieve whatever you set your mind on doing. You can live an authentic life—where your actions are aligned with your beliefs and values. Where time flies because you're in "the zone" as you do the things that you love.

Anyone who has ever competed in or watched an athletic race has seen how the athlete—as much as he or she might have struggled during the race—can somewhere from deep within draw upon the last bit of strength to triumphantly sprint (I prefer "fly") across the finish line. It's a moment of triumph, empowerment, and inspiration to be cherished. Learn to take flight yourself!

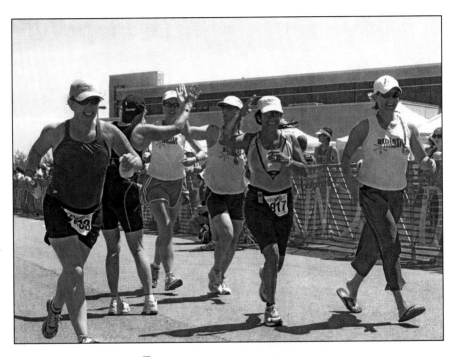

FRIENDS AT THE FINISH LINE
(PHOTO COURTESY OF BRIGHTROOM.COM)

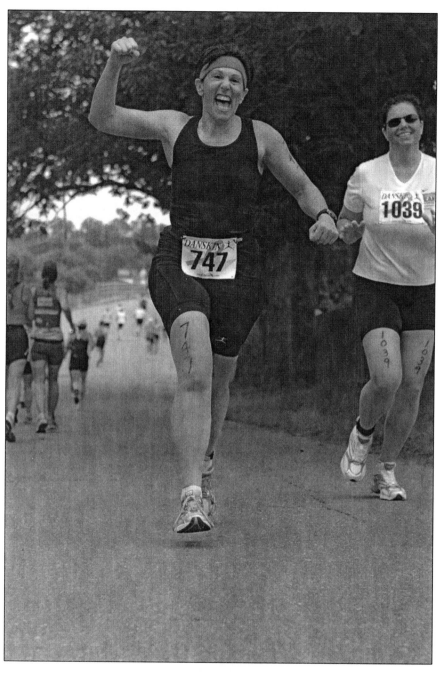

TRIATHLETE JODI KAPLAN
(PHOTO COURTESY OF BRIGHTROOM.COM)

CHAPTER 2

Being Authentically You

> *"Today I stand a little taller and walk a little prouder because I am a triathlete. I was invincible and unstoppable—suddenly I could fly."*
> – Lisa Soler

As women, we are pulled in a multitude of directions in our lives… family, career, friends, hobbies, volunteer opportunities, self-care and health, etc. Plus we try to meet the expectations of others around us. Because it's so easy to get consumed with meeting all these competing demands, it's essential that we take time out *on purpose* to listen to ourselves. Otherwise, we can easily lose sight of who we truly are.

LESSON: Take a look at who you are and who you want to be. Create the life you dream of.

In order to live authentically, we need to create a life that is in line with what's important to us. When our living feels out of alignment with our real self, getting back on track can take some sorting through.

REALIZING DREAMS
by Carmen Guy

"Team Dream, Team Dream, Team Dream." That's all I heard my non-athletic, belly-dancing friend talk about for a whole year! Deciding to try something new, she joined Team Dream, a triathlon team for women of color. This group of women—who come in all sizes and athletic abilities—inspired her so much, she wanted to share her experience with the world.

Breaking all stereotypes about the sport, these women have some things in common. They enjoying learning "to raise their game" (the team motto) through coaching and information to keep themselves physically active and emotionally fit.

Unlike my formerly non-athletic friend, I learned at a young age that physical activities can provide the motivation needed to raise self-esteem. As a result of my love for physical activities, I pursued my degree in physical education, but I stopped being active after college. Even though I am a Physical Education teacher, I told my students what to do instead of showing them. Weight gain, a sedentary lifestyle, and some health issues had me coaching from the sidelines instead of being actively involved in sports.

But the more I learned about this triathlon team, the more I wanted in. I asked myself. *Can I do this?* I was 51, overweight, had high blood pressure and artificial hips on both sides. *Should I dare to dream?* I thought to myself. *Was it crazy to want back what I loved so much—to be an active participant?* It was time for my visit to the doctor to see how well the second hip was holding up. He said I was doing fine, and suggested I start an exercise program. So, imagine my shock when he suggested swimming, walking and biking. It was my dream made to order. As the kids at school would say, I was "thirsty" (wanting something so badly) because I wanted to be a Team Dreamer. It didn't help that I was really jealous of my friend who had turned into an athlete. I'll never forget the day she opened up her trunk to put something in and I saw a gym bag and a bike. "Oh, my God! You really are an athlete." *I* was helping *her* shop for athletic gear.

I soon found out joining was the *easy* part. As a member of Team Dream, our main goal was to participate in the Chicagoland Danskin triathlon. As I pushed myself to train, I also joined Weight Watchers and I lost 50 pounds.

A couple of weeks before the Danskin, my former non-athletic friend gave me a book titled *Slow Fat Triathlete*. At first I refused to read it because I really didn't want to read about a slow, fat woman. Reluctantly, I began to read the book and loved it. So I had to admit that my friend was right again. This book was and is my bible and my inspiration.

Registration time came for the Danskin and I had not mastered the bike. So, after much debate, I decided that the first year I would compete on a relay team doing the swim and the 5k. I didn't know if I could handle all three with not one, but two titanium hips! The day of the race arrived, and I noticed something right away. Besides there being so many women in one place, I also noticed the atmosphere. I think Danskin must give every participant a checklist on what to bring to the race: a big smile, lots of laughter, a unity, a positive attitude, and celebration of every success.

As I neared the end of my race, I thought of the changes that had taken place—my new attitude and fitness level. Before the Danskin I couldn't walk a block, but I crossed the finish line last year and I can't wait to do it again this year. Thanks Team Dream for being a builder of dreams.

Carmen Guy is a physical education teacher, and when she's not training for a triathlon, she's doing as many 5k races as she can find. The story of her formerly non-athletic friend, Stephanie, follows later in the chapter.

BECOMING AN IRON(WO)MAN TRIATHLETE
by Annette Jonker

How did all of this start? Six years ago, I was climbing the corporate ladder, doing well, but realizing that there might be more to life than work. I knew life could have been worse, but I also thought it could be better.

Looking back, I realize that I'd gone through the same lifestyle changes that most people do over time. In primary school, I was extremely active. I loved swimming, played outside, enjoyed sports and even cycled to school. Throughout high school, as I got older, I became less active. Since high school was a bus journey away, my bike was stashed in the garage to collect cobwebs.

In college, sports were for people who were good at it. I wasn't very athletic so the thought of participating didn't even cross my mind. My first years at work were all about proving myself: working really hard and long hours didn't leave time for much else.

It happened gradually over time, but I found myself overweight and sedentary. I started going to the gym and set a goal to work out three times a week. I always thought it was really unfair that some people can eat what they want, work out a little, and not gain any weight. I was not so lucky. I now realize that this is partly myth and potentially genetic.

I moved to Chicago and, though working out three times a week had stuck, I needed a bit more of a challenge. A group of us were chatting when my friend, Amy, mentioned that she'd heard of the Danskin triathlon and thought that we should all sign up. To say that I had reservations is an understatement. I had never heard of triathlon and didn't believe that I could do it. Amy went on a crusade to get everyone signed up. Those she first convinced tried to persuade the rest of us. They were determined and I finally caved in. If they were going to try, I would too.

We started training together and I found it was much easier to get to the gym with a goal in mind and friends waiting. Most of us started out not able to run for more than three minutes, let alone 3 miles. It was challenging, but we all got to the point where we could walk/run the 3 miles. It felt great. I also loved being on a bike and riding like a kid. There was a shift in my attitude. I expected more from life.

During that time, I came to the realization that I really wasn't happy at work. Climbing the corporate ladder, I had reached a point where I needed to either fight to get to the next rung or change course. I decided to change course, resigned and took some time off. I'd always wanted to travel through East Africa so off I went.

It was a great trip but unfortunately, timing-wise, this decision meant that I missed doing the triathlon I had trained for with my friends. Upon my return, I heard all about how much fun they had, how inspired they felt and how supportive all of the other triathletes were. Everyone was pleased that they had successfully completed their first triathlon and planned to do it again the following year. I realized that I wanted to join them and made the commitment.

As time went by, I started getting more and more into fitness and decided to focus on losing some weight. As I lost weight, I gained confidence. As I got fitter, it became less of a struggle to run and, believe me, losing 40 pounds made a HUGE difference in how comfortable I felt running. I did a couple of 5k races, but it was the thought of doing the Danskin with my friends that kept me going.

I did my first Danskin in 2004. I went for body markings (before the start of the race where your race number is written on you) and the guy with the Sharpie said he needed to write on my "biceps." I was shocked, my arms had never been called that—I didn't even think I had those… biceps… cool… I have biceps.

In 2004, when I became a triathlete, I was still smoking a pack a day. At least I had taken the first couple of steps toward fitness. I later quit smoking because I realized that I couldn't expect to get any better at running if I was still smoking. Three days after I quit, I ran 3.5 miles without stopping; running had never felt so good. That's one of the runs I know I will always remember.

Three years later, I was privileged to be a Workout Leader for Team Danskin Training in Chicago. It was great seeing women just like me starting out and completing their first triathlon. It was a gratifying experience to provide a support infrastructure and be someone that they could turn to.

I've been really fortunate and, with some encouragement and a lot of training, I completed my first Ironman in 2007. I still can't believe it. It was one of the best days of my life. Four years earlier, I could barely run. Now I'm contemplating doing my second Iron-distance race. I still ride my bike like I did in primary school. I'm fitter now than I was in high school. Doing triathlons makes me feel like a kid again and I love it!

I decided to part ways with the corporate world for now and focus on triathlon coaching: the sense of satisfaction I gain from training people is amazing. I've noticed the change in my life. It's not that I felt bad before, but being fit feels awesome.

Fitness has become my life. I've joined Sally Edwards' quest to help get America fit and hope to contribute by coaching and encouraging people to get involved with triathlon. I want to continue to swim, bike and run and encourage you to do the same.

Triathlon is a race involving a lot of people. For most of us, the competition is between "me now" and "me last year"—not each other. Whatever happens, I know that just by becoming a triathlete, I've won.

Annette Jonker lives in Chicago and started My Fitness Company, LLC to encourage people to tri and reach their potential. She is a native of South Africa.

Who you are today is a function of the talents and skills you possess—*your strengths*—as well as the vast experiences of your past. One way to find clues for getting back in touch with your true self is to think about activities you enjoyed in your youth. What you enjoyed as a child will be different from the next woman. For you, it might have been playing the piano; for another woman, artwork may have consumed her extra hours. In terms of exercise, perhaps you loved to dance, whereas your sister often went skating.

Both Carmen and Annette re-created their lives in ways that make them feel good about who they are and what they're doing. They looked back and identified activities that made them happy in their earlier days—and in both cases, this was *physical activity*. For Carmen, that was the reason she became a PE teacher. For Annette, the bike rides and physical activity of her elementary school days brought joy.

Carmen had many reasons for why she found herself in an unsatisfactory place before deciding to train for her first Danskin triathlon. She was overweight and sedentary and had gone through two hip replacements. Fresh perspectives, including encouragement from her friend Stephanie, allowed her to change the interpretation of those facts. No longer did she have to accept being too heavy and inactive. Carmen created a new way of living based on activity and physical fitness, and she was able to accomplish things she had previously thought unachievable.

Annette was so determined to live an authentic life that she left the corporate world to pursue her growing interest in triathlon. She became a much healthier, happier person, someone who substantially raised the bar by training for and completing an Ironman triathlon. Annette also discovered her love of triathlon coaching. She is spending time now on things that really matter to her, feeling good about who she is.

LESSON: Accept who you are, as you are. Don't be your own worst critic.

As women, we are often our own harshest critics. But what if we gave ourselves the same compassion and consideration that we would extend to our best friend? We need to start being kinder to and more understanding of ourselves. Then, after letting go of our negativity and also accepting who we are, we can move our lives forward in a positive direction.

IT STARTED WITH A BRA
by Stephanie Gates

All my life my body has been a mixed blessing because of the attention—positive and negative—it brings from people. More introverted than extroverted, I haven't always known how to handle the attention. You see, I'm a Barbie with a booty. This makes me self-conscious at times. On top of that, I'm clumsy; so like many women, I don't always love the skin I'm in.

Who would have thought that a conversation about a bra would be the catalyst I needed to change my life? It was the summer, and I had just finished a grueling workout with a personal trainer. I was trying to will my spaghetti legs to carry me home when the conversation in the locker room turned to sports bras. I almost laughed out loud—to keep from crying. I know why Barbie has everything but a good bra. They're hard as hell to find! And sports bras are out of the question.

But this woman seemed to know a lot about bras, so I listened. When I bought my Enell sports bra, life got *so* much better. For the first time since elementary school, I was able to run and jump without incident. Then the bra lady told me about a women-of-color triathlon team. Me? Triathlons were long, grueling races for White men. How was I, a 40-year-old Black woman, going to finish a triathlon? Swim? Loved water, but was afraid of the deep end of the pool. Bike? On the lake front with my friends at a leisurely pace, and I stress leisurely! Run? Away from gym class in grammar school and two years of torture in high school, until I escaped to modern dance. With all of the reasons not to check it out, I thought, *Why not check it out?*

The first meeting was in October, and though I had tried to recruit some friends, only one went with me to the meeting. She left; I stayed and stepped into a surreal experience. The energy was incredible; I felt charged and encouraged as myths and stereotypes about triathlon dissipated that day. It was not for White men only, but any woman who dared to try. I realized that women are not always catty—we can show love and support for one another. Also, age was not a factor as the oldest woman in the room was in her 70s. It was as though I was outside of myself looking, listening, and feeling as these women shared their stories of triathlon and triumph. I signed up and later talked my sister-in-law into joining.

When training season started, I was in a funk. On the out-side things looked good, but inside I was hurting and I didn't know how to stop the hurt. Change had moved into my house and rearranged it, and I was having a hard time adjusting. When I was alone, I cried constantly. To make matters worse,

I felt bad about feeling bad. I had family, friends, a job, good health, and few worries, but there was little joy in my life.

Training was the exception. I was learning so much—about the sport, about my teammates, about myself. I signed up for everything—circuit training, bike development, and swimming. Many days I was tired and frustrated because I didn't think I was progressing fast enough, forgetting it was my first year. But I kept going. I had anxiety about the water as the numbers in swim class dwindled, but I stuck to it and my teammates kept me encouraged.

One day after swim, I had an amazing shift in my thinking. Prior to becoming a triathlete, I didn't like changing my clothes in front of people. It was the whole body image thing. But on this day, as we laughed, talked and showered, sharing shampoo and soap, I looked at the women on my team through different eyes. I saw bodies that had birthed life, nursed life, been knocked down by life but were still standing strong. These women had stepped outside of their ordinary existence to do extraordinary things. The scars, stretch marks and cellulite that marked our collective bodies showed real life, and not some airbrushed version. Every naked body in the locker room was beautiful!

Talking myself out of the swim, I signed up to be a part of a relay team my first year. At first I felt bad but then I thought, *There's always next year.* The morning of the Danskin gave me chills. Not only was I in the company of my teammates, but thousands of other women who dared to "tri." It was the same camaraderie and sisterhood that I felt with fellow dreamers, but tenfold!

As I waited for my swimmer to come out of the water so I could jump on the bike and get in the race, I saw them lift a woman out of the water and put her in a wheelchair to begin the second leg of the triathlon. My breath froze in my chest.

At that moment, I knew something greater than myself was at work. Though I cry tears of pain, I seldom cry tears of joy. But when I got on my bike, I began to cry, but stopped because I had a race to finish. I knew that my life had changed—for the better and there was no turning back.

Stephanie Gates is an elementary school librarian. In addition to being a triathlete, Stephanie is a writer, belly dancer and avid reader.

IN AN INSTANT...
by Susanne Achtenhagen

Sixteen years ago, I did my first triathlon. I was in college, had learned about the three-sport adventure, and was curious. I grew up swimming, ran on the beach in Santa Barbara where I was in school, and certainly knew how to ride a bike. I finished my first race third in my age group and was hooked.

Throughout the 1990s, I trained and raced. I realized more than ever that training was a way to get me out of my head, stop my thinking, and help me enjoy the outdoors. I also liked the benefits of how my body looked and the attention I got for my long tan legs.

Over the years, I trained more and raced longer. I had a goal of racing in the Ironman Hawaii one day, never before having swum 2.4 miles, ridden 112 or run 26. Over time I prepared for and accomplished each of those distances to where in 1998, I signed up for Ironman Canada. My training took a great deal of my time. I worked, trained and ate.

With the increase in training, I was able to eat a ton of food and "get away with it." Over time, food and exercise were the only ways I knew how to calm myself. They were the answer to everything in my life. If I was sad, I ran and ate. If

I needed company, I rode and ate. These were the "healthy" choices.

I always said I could never be anorexic because I liked food too much. Never say never. I continued to train a ton and started eating almost nothing. I got down to a weight that was much too light for me. I loved all of the positive comments I received; they fueled me and I thrived on them. I had no ability to see myself as worthy and loveable as I was so I lived for comments from the outside.

Three years ago, my world changed. After 12 years of struggling to find my own happiness, a single question changed everything.

"What if you were okay just as you are today?" a friend asked.

In an instant, everything changed. I had been living as a self-defined "sick" person trying to get healthy. For nearly 20 years, I had struggled, believing I had an eating disorder (anorexia/bulimia/excess exercise). Suddenly, I saw myself as a healthy person trying to live the best life possible.

My world changed because my thinking changed. Old habits fell away like leaves in the wind. And I realized that change, *all* change, requires one simple thing: that we change our minds. No longer spending massive amounts of time and energy trying to fix my life, I was finally free to live an inspired life.

One year ago, I decided to act. As the 35-year-old mother of two girls, I decided to compete as a triathlete again. I had some unfinished business that I needed to address: could I be a great triathlete? In the past year, inspired by a clear vision, I qualified as a professional triathlete.

Ultimately, I want to compete in the 2008 Olympics.

My vision, however, goes beyond even the Olympics. Because I have experienced personally the transformative power of a new thought, I want to use my life as a triathlete and mother as a metaphor to inspire people to change their thinking, to discover new perspectives on health and well-being, and to follow their dreams.

Triathlon is the venue I am choosing to get my face, my voice, and my vision of health and well-being into the world. I hope that being a wife, mother of two, and successful triathlete will inspire people to explore new ways of thinking, living and being.

Susanne Achtenhagen lives in Boulder, Colorado with her husband and two beautiful daughters. Her website is www.triathletemom.com.

Our interpretations of the experiences we have help define who we are—for the good and the bad. Fortunately, negative perspectives can change for the better over time. As we have new experiences, the facts of our lives change, and we can gain more confidence and a sense of pride in ourselves. Fresh perspectives and priorities allow us to look back and put new interpretations on our history.

Based on her life experiences, Stephanie hadn't come to terms with who she is—she wasn't comfortable in her own skin because of her abundant "booty." This is a woman who didn't believe she was an athlete and certainly not a triathlete. Her life held little joy or happiness. But when she discovered triathlon and Team Dream, Stephanie woke up to an exciting possibility. And as she pursued this unlikely path, Stephanie found a place where she could grow and learn. Then suddenly, one day when Stephanie was with her teammates, she changed the interpretation of the facts of her life. No longer was she uncomfortable with her body. Stephanie began to appreciate who she is. It happened in an instant with just a change in her way of thinking.

Susanne's experience was much the same, as she too needed to come to terms with herself. Physical fitness had been a priority in her life for years. However, in Susanne's mind, she used physical fitness and her appearance as a crutch to compensate for her own insecurities. She was hard on herself mentally and beat herself up as she struggled with her weight and anorexia and bulimia issues. However, when challenged by her friend's question (*"What if you were okay just as you are today?"*), Susanne was suddenly able to change the interpretation of the facts of her life. She began to view physical fitness as a *positive force* in her life. Susanne finally let go of the mental anguish related to eating. Her mind and body became connected. She was then able to create a life that was full of positive energy.

LESSON: You deserve a high ranking on your own priority list. Besides, you can take better care of others when you first take care of yourself.

As women, we are life's primary caregivers. We readily put the needs of our families and others first. As a result, our own needs can easily end up at the bottom of the priority list. Though we may think of taking time for ourselves as "selfish," it is anything but. When we give more to ourselves, we experience joy and feel happier. Then we have more to give to those around us.

WHAT A "NEW NORMAL" MEANT
by Jodi Kaplan

I have been an athlete all of my life. I always enjoyed participating in team sports. But if someone told me a year ago that I was going to be a triathlete, I would have told them that they are absolutely crazy. Lots of things were different one year ago—even six months ago.

February 1, 2006 is the day that life changed. My husband was diagnosed with glioblastoma, a form of brain cancer. What that meant for us, we didn't know, but we knew our lives would never be the same. No one knows how they will react to devastating news like this until they are actually faced with it. We surprised ourselves and continue to do so. We realized that we had to change our perceptions of normalcy—we live a "new normal" now.

In the midst of this life-changing experience, I met a wonderful woman who also was dealing with glioblastoma in her family. In a crazy twist of fate, we learned that we actually share a cousin. I guess we were supposed to meet. It turns out that she was recruiting women for the Danskin Triathlon. I took her card, but didn't really believe that I would be able to compete in a triathlon. My curiosity got the best of me and I went to the website. Once I began reading, I was hooked. There was a team involved and I always loved team sports! The thought of being on a team that was being coached was very attractive to me. I was living that new normal and I needed some time to focus on me. I spoke to my husband about it and he was incredibly supportive. He knew that this would help me both emotionally and physically.

The experience was amazing. I did things that I never thought I could do. During our first training session, I could hardly run 1.5 miles. Just a few months later, I was able to run

4 miles. I was certainly not breaking any speed records, but I was able to do it and I was getting better and better. The team was phenomenal, everyone was so supportive. I met some very cool women who were like me—a mother, wife, daughter, sister, employee. We get pulled in every direction and there is no time for ourselves. This made me make time for myself.

Crossing the finish line brought a rash of emotions, the tears were streaming. This was a great accomplishment for me: way out of my comfort zone, empowering, satisfying and invigorating. I felt so proud that I set this stretch goal and achieved it. My husband shared this pride in my accomplishment. My children (ages 9 and 11) picked up some great messages as well. My 9-year-old daughter is planning to compete in a Danskin triathlon with me when she turns 14. I have not stopped my training. Since the Danskin, I have done another triathlon and a road race.

I am going to continue to sign up for races throughout the year so that I am motivated to train. I cannot lose the momentum that the Danskin Triathlon has started... it has truly been a valuable experience for my emotional and physical well-being. You don't know if you don't tri!

Jodi Kaplan completed her first Danskin in Webster, Massachusetts in 2006 and improved her time by 8 minutes for her second Danskin in 2007. After submitting her initial story, Jodi provided an update. "February 1st is Steve's two-year anniversary since diagnosis. Steve is beating the odds! I believe that a positive attitude does help to fight illness and Steve is proof of that. There is certainly reason to celebrate!"

NO LONGER LAST ON THE LIST
by Stacy Roberts

I heard about the Danskin from a few of my friends who had participated in it last year. I decided to make the commitment to myself as a New Year's resolution to live a healthier lifestyle. I didn't even own a bike at the time and life's excuses seemed to have prevented me from truly focusing on my body and healthy exercise. My idea of swimming was taking my two boys to the lake and reading a magazine while watching them play. And running is something I hadn't done since grade school while playing Kiss Or Kill on the playground. Basically, I made the commitment with no knowledge of what I was getting into. What I did know was that I needed something.

I am an office manager at an elementary school and between caring for 400 students and 60 staff all day long, then coming home and managing my household and providing a healthy balanced life for my children, I'm exhausted. Time is minimal for myself and often my personal desires are last on the list of priorities.

Knowing that I knew nothing and was going to need assistance, I signed up to train with the TriBabes of Seattle, Washington. I am forever grateful for Coach Lisa Ballou and the TriBabes for the incredible knowledge and inspiration they shared with me. I will admit, I still used my excuses during the week and didn't always complete my training schedule. But every Saturday morning, at the team training meetings, I challenged my body and grew wiser as a woman. Watching and participating with woman of all ages, sizes and shapes grew a part of me that will forever shine. My life has been changed.

As I trained for the Danskin, the focus was always on me. I didn't think about cancer or the fight for its cure. But on race day, I was overcome with emotions. I had lost a best friend in

February 2006 to cancer and participating with cancer survivors and observing 5,000 women coming together to fight cancer brought an incredible sense of meaning into my heart. There were times during the swim when I sucked in so much water I thought I was going to drown. There was a time on my bike when I witnessed a woman flip head over her handle bars and thought, *Please God, don't let me run her over.* There was a time while I was running and my feet were so numb I wasn't sure I was moving. But every time I was challenged, I continued and I told myself "yes." *Yes, you can do it. You are doing it. It can be done.* Flying over the finish line brings new life. Come fly with me next year, I will be there!

Stacy Roberts, 38, is a single mother of two boys, Cody (11) and Conner (9). Stacy dedicates her story to the memory of her dear friend, Lisa Campos, who passed away from cancer on February 13, 2006, and to Lisa's two children, Kristine and Robbie.

When life's many priorities push us around, it's easy not to recognize that the person holding us back from a better experience is truly ourselves. We need to decide to give ourselves time, care, compassion and fun.

When Stacy decided to do something for herself by training for a Danskin triathlon, she had a wonderful experience that inspired her. Aside from the satisfaction of the activity and the support of the team meetings, the exercise created new energy in her life. Long gone were the days when exercise meant taking her two boys to the lake and reading magazines while they swam. With the experience of flying over the finish line came a new commitment—to continue to make time for this new interest that gave back so much to her life.

Jodi undoubtedly benefited from the positive aspects—both physical and psychological—that result from regular, vigorous exercise. As a result, she was better able to handle the extreme stress that accompanied her husband's health diagnosis. Jodi's triathlon training forced her to take care of herself first—at least some of the time. Her husband and family benefited from Jodi's time away since she was better able to handle the emotions and requirements that came with their situation.

LESSON: Live your dreams and uncover the authentic you. Live an empowered life!

Empowerment has been defined as a feeling of personal control over all domains of our lives. It allows us a sense of our own value and strength and the ability to handle life's problems. Empowerment taps into the potential that exists within each one of us, providing self-confidence and self-esteem.

THE ROAD TO MY FIRST DANSKIN
by Ruth Kaminski

I am the poster child for unlikely athletes. I'm older, not fast, not graceful, and spandex is NOT my friend. These may sound like negative statements, but the reality is they are facts. I accept them and embrace them because I no longer allow these things to stop me.

There are times in our lives when we can clearly see our roles change and we redefine who we are and how we think of ourselves. Looking back, I see reaching the age of majority and putting childhood behind me, becoming a wife and then a mother, the arrival of my grandchildren. I thought that my shining moments of epic events were past me... until, at the age of 50, I became a triathlete. Just saying that gives me the chills and a secret smile on my face!

In 2005, I was feeling like something was missing in my life. I had two very serious back surgeries in July 2002 and the road back was proving to be very long and painful. Most activities were difficult for me to do, but I was feeling the need to do something! So I joined a deep-water aerobics class. I really enjoyed it and discovered that moving my body seemed to be adding a missing piece to my happiness. Then I met a woman who said she was going to do a triathlon. I told her I would cheer her on and I tried to sound positive as I was thinking she had to be crazy! Why would anyone want to do such a thing? Well, those were my famous "last thoughts" because somehow she got me to agree that I could join a relay team and do a part of a triathlon. She told me about a group of women who were getting together for one sole purpose—to train for, encourage each other, and complete the 2005 Danskin Triathlon in Seattle. There were nine of us, all middle-aged and not in athletic condition. Each of us was either still overweight then or had been in the recent past. But there we were... "The Women of Substance" group was born!

Slowly training began: swimming, biking, and running/walking. My plan was to do the 3.1-mile walk. I was sure that wouldn't put too much strain on my still-healing back... besides, I was positive I would drown if I tried to swim a half mile and biking 12 was a feat beyond imagination! So I found another person, and did the same thing done to me... I had her agreeing to do the bike portion of a triathlon before she realized what happened to her. Like the majority of the group, she had never dreamed of doing a triathlon or any major sporting event.

At first I made excuses to not make it to training events. I was terrified of this commitment I made. I was not positive that I would really follow through on this, so I was stockpiling my excuses. I analyzed every little ache and pain—was I doing damage to this old, out-of-shape body? But as the pains passed

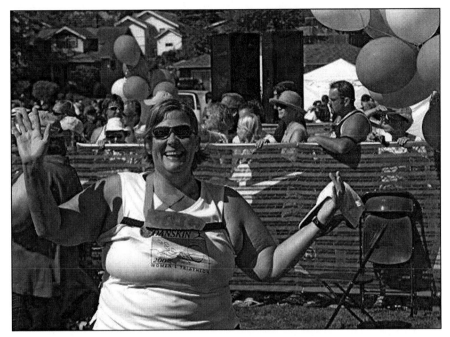

TRIATHLETE RUTH KAMINSKI

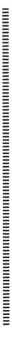

and then actually diminished in their appearances, I had to admit it was just my muscles learning to work again. So I began showing up more. One day I realized that while we were working out, and definitely getting fitter, we also were supporting each other emotionally. We spent a good deal of every workout laughing. It dawned on me that I was having FUN! Instead of making excuses, or showing up to train because the others expected me, I eagerly showed up and even began additional training on my own.

I hadn't found someone to do the swim portion, and as the training went further, I realized that I wanted to do more. I decided secretly that I would do the swim AND the run/walk... that is, IF I actually followed through on this. At some point, the desire to do the triathlon was overcoming my fear of failure. But I knew that to truly become committed I needed to start "being" an athlete, and that meant openly telling family and friends I was training for an event. Once I said it—put it out there—I knew I would *have* to do the triathlon to save face.

I told my adult daughters first. They said all the right words but I could hear the disbelief and amusement in their tones. My 19-year-old son just looked at me as if I had lost my mind and said, "Whatever, Mom." I was used to being their "crazy mom," and I knew that they would be supportive. I did not tell my husband I had signed up to do the Danskin until I had a couple of months' training under my belt. My husband is one of those natural athletes, and works hard to stay fit and in shape. I was afraid he would laugh at me or tell me that I couldn't do it. Instead, he got on the support bandwagon. He worked out with me, lowering his pace to meet mine, then was surprised and delighted when my pace increased. Emboldened, I told my co-workers what I was doing. Now that admission got open laughter and disbelief! Everyone involved, myself included, was really wondering if I would follow through, if I would really do this.

As the months went by, my confidence increased. Instead of hiding under layers of sweat clothes on my way to do open-water swims in the lake, I courageously walked around in my skintight triathlon suit. Now, that takes guts to be an old, fat woman walking around in spandex in public! I was evolving into an athlete. A month before the Danskin, we decided to bolster our courage and do the entire distance, all three legs with the transitions. All I can say is WOW! It was hard, it was long, it was tiring, and I had never had so much fun in my whole life!!!

One thing though was still terrifying me. How would I have enough courage to actually participate in an athletic event? I had never done that. A couple of weeks before the Danskin, there was an Iron Girl 5K run/walk. I registered for the race. I told no one… I didn't even tell my husband until the morning of the event. I refused to allow anyone to accompany me in case I humiliated myself. I just needed to see how it would feel to race, to see how I felt as I was passed and left far behind, how I would feel if I was last. Once I crossed that finish line, *not last by the way*, I knew that I would be OK at the Danskin.

The Danskin Triathlon itself was incredible. What they say is true: the woman that finishes the race is not the same woman who started. I'm not going to lie, right up until the time you actually start swimming, it is scary. But then your body just does what you've taught it to do. Spectators, other athletes, volunteers cheer you on and in return you cheer them on and then you cross the finish line and it's over. You shed many tears of joy and excitement and feel so incredible that you did something that you never thought you could and you absolutely cannot wait to do it again! At that moment, you realize… I am an athlete!

I want to let everyone know that if they want to do this, they can. It's about finishing, it's about overcoming fears, it's about allowing yourself to rise up to your own expectations and secret dreams. Making sure you train in all events is crucial, because it is a guarantee for success if your body can go into autopilot when the fear is at its highest. Learn from the experts—Sally Edwards' books were invaluable, also John Bingham's books provided inspiration. Find people to train with. I can't tell you how far it moves you along when you have someone looking you in the eye, lying through their teeth, telling you that you look beautiful in spandex so quit whining and get moving! Find a mantra that you can hold on to, to help you hope when believing is hard. My mantra shifted as the need arose. The one that stuck, though, was the one that developed when I was scared witless, embarrassed by my age, size and thoughts that I just couldn't do this. It was: *I CAN do this; one step at a time!*

I did fly across the finish line last year, but it was the soaring and dancing of my spirit rather than the fleetness of my feet. I have a long way to go before this will become second nature to me. I do know that I'm having fun, and borrowing an image from Jeff Lynne and Tom Petty, I am learning to fly without wings. So crank up the stereo on "Learning to Fly" by Tom Petty and Heartbreakers, dance around your living room, and come fly with me!

Ruth Kaminski lives in Seattle, Washington and is a member of Women of Substance. In addition to being the mother of three, she has four grandchildren. Every few years, she likes to do something out of the character to "shake things up"—which may explain her two tattoos, shaving her head (to benefit a charity), and becoming a triathlete.

THE TRANSFORMATION OF MY SISTER, LISA
by Janine Santacroce

My sister Lisa was turning 40 and it was her personal goal to finish the Danskin triathlon.

Years ago, when Lisa was 19, she had thyroid cancer. After the diagnosis, never looking back, she faced the cancer head-on. She had surgery to remove a tumor the size of a softball, neck tissue and her thyroid. Left with a scar across her entire neck, she never felt sorry for herself as she fought cancer. At times, she held our family together. Fifteen years later after giving birth to her son, the cancer returned. With the same strength and courage, she had treatment and once again fought off the cancer.

When registering for the race, on the form was a box, "Check here if you are a cancer survivor." Lisa had never acknowledged being a cancer survivor, never would bring attention to herself or the accomplishments in her life. She is an intelligent, beautiful, generous, kind soul who would give you the shirt off her back. But she was always standing on the sidelines supporting everyone else, never believing in her own strength or taking the time to fulfill her own dreams.

When completing the Danskin registration form, Lisa checked off "cancer survivor"—acknowledging for the first time that being a cancer survivor is part of who she is.

For both Lisa and me, crossing the finish line changed our lives. Next to giving birth to our children, it was the most powerful thing we had ever done.

After the race, I received a letter from Lisa. She wrote:

Today I stand a little taller and walk a little prouder because I am a triathlete. The moment my feet touched the sand after the swim, tears rolled down my cheeks and the biggest smile crossed my face. I felt liberated and filled with a sense of accomplishment. By the time I was on my bike, I was not the same person. I was invincible and unstoppable—suddenly I could fly.

When it came to the run, I was strong and powerful. With the finish line in sight, every emotion filled my body and my eyes once again filled with tears. I can't think of a better way to start celebrating the next milestone of my "NEW" life—not "MID" life—than crossing the finish line of a triathlon with my best friend, my sister.

Janine Santacroce and her sister Lisa Soler completed their first Danskin at Sandy Hook, New Jersey. They returned the following year, having recruited additional friends to join them.

Crossing the finish line of a triathlon is often described as "life-changing" and "empowering." After spending time training for an event that sometimes seems only possible in her dreams, the triathlete learns that if she can accomplish this, she can achieve whatever she sets her minds on doing. She may discover strengths she never knew existed and find that she has an "inner athlete" waiting to get out.

Ruth, Janine and Lisa all experienced the power of the finish line. They tapped into potential that existed inside each one of them.

It wasn't until Lisa reached the age of 40 that she discovered untapped aspects of her personal strength. Although she had courageously faced two battles with cancer, Lisa was not aware of much of her own potential. That is, until she completed her first triathlon alongside her sister Janine. Lisa was transformed from shy and reserved to confident and powerful.

As with Lisa, triathlon was a catalyst for change and empowerment for Ruth. Instead of shyness, Ruth's challenge was overcoming her self-limiting beliefs about what a 50-year-old should and shouldn't do. Training for her first triathlon allowed Ruth to explode those myths. For both Lisa and Ruth, flying over the finish line in their first triathlons was a redefining moment in their lives.

Consider the experience of Danskin participant Kathy Pulda:

"The Danskin has been a life-changing event for me. Now having finished my second one at age 54, I know I can do anything I set my mind on doing. It gave me the confidence I needed last year, when I returned to graduate school to get my master's [degree] in nursing, with women young enough to be my daughters. If I could do the Danskin, I could succeed in graduate school."

Take Stock and Find the "Authentic You"

Getting to a place of overwhelm doesn't happen overnight. As a number of the stories in this chapter illustrate, none of the women gained the extra 40 or 50 pounds in a week or two. But a few pounds a year over a number of years all add up. So it is with our lives more generally. We may start out with jobs after graduation. Add a spouse, some kids, a house, a dog, etc.—or whatever has been tacked on and combined in your life. One day you wake up and realize your time is all divvied up and you're not leading the life you desire.

Take time now to stop and get acquainted again with the real you. Don't wait for a life-changing event, such as an illness or death of someone you love, to force you to make changes. Look to your past to determine who you are—your "old story." Along with this, identify the old perceptions and beliefs that are holding you back. Let them go! Then look forward and think about who you want to be in your life and how you want that life to look.

Make a commitment to yourself TODAY! Do something *for you*. Make some important changes, even if they're baby steps at first. Figure out who you are and where you want to go. And then do it!

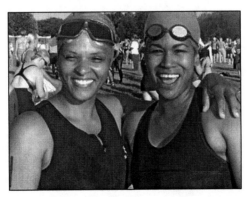

TEAM DREAM MEMBERS
DARLENE DENNARD AND ELAINE ELAM

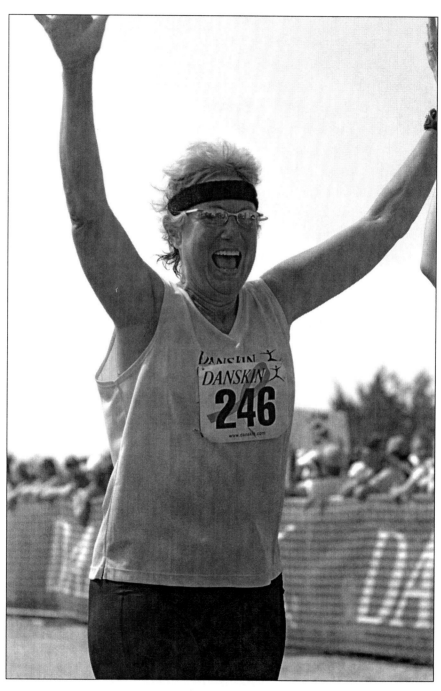

Dianne Michaels completes her journey.
(photo courtesy of brightroom.com)

CHAPTER 3

She Who Has the Most Fun Wins!

(In other words, Success is how YOU define it.)

> *"I'm too old and too smart and too accomplished to let anybody define success for me but myself."*
> – Anna Quinlan

Although thousands of women complete the Danskin and other triathlons each year, their reasons and motivations for doing so are varied. Ultimately, every woman must personally define what successful participation will mean to her. In the same way, the definition of what constitutes success in achieving *any* goal will also depend on the individual. There is virtually no right or wrong definition of "success."

For a lot of the Danskin women—many of whom never set an athletic goal before this triathlon—success means crossing the finish line in whatever time it takes. Or success may be completing one leg of the triathlon (swim, bike, run/walk) as part of a relay team. Meanwhile, on the same course, there are elite athletes competing to be the top finisher. Others are racing against themselves to create a new "PB" (personal best) compared to results of a previous year at the Danskin or at a different triathlon. For others still, it's all about learning from the journey.

As Lynn Sparks of Austin, Texas (a three-time previous Danskin participant) said, "On race day, I get to set my own pace... even if there does seem to be an undercurrent of 'beat your last time.' I just want to finish and be proud of myself for it."[10]

LESSON: Our lives contain a multitude of choices. Only *you* can make the decisions that are right for you to create your own definition of success.

One advantage of being female is that we have plenty of choices. Celebrate this fact by making the choices that are right for you in terms of what constitutes a successful life. Our days are full of options.

When you choose to get back to physical activity, there are plenty of benefits (more on this back in Chapter 1). Therefore, being fit should be a priority in your life. Regular, vigorous exercise will improve your mental capacity and bring you peace of mind. It will keep you active, agile and energetic even as you age. However, the way you decide to exercise up to you.

If you decide to do an athletic event, whether it be a Danskin triathlon or some other experience, congratulate yourself just for being there—*however you participate*. Enjoy the experience on your own terms and have fun!

A NEW OUTLET FOR MY INNER ATHLETE
by Betsy Oudenhoven

I have always considered myself an athlete; however, I was not a triathlete until I completed my first Danskin sprint triathlon right before my 49th birthday. I never planned to do a triathlon. I wasn't sure I could. As a working mother and marathoner, I couldn't imagine where people found the time to train for three sports. Plus there was the problem of swimming. I learned to swim in Lake Ontario when I was a kid, but that was many years and very few swimsuits ago. It just wasn't something I continued into my adult life. So, happy on dry land, I never gave triathlons much thought.

But then, like many older runners, knee problems motivated me to join a cycling class where I could get a good workout and get off my feet. I had only been spinning for a few months when a couple of the women in my class began talking about doing the Danskin triathlon in Wisconsin in July. I was intrigued. I learned that there was a "sprint" distance and that you could do any swim stroke you wanted (I thought there was a rule that you had to do freestyle). I also loved the fact that it was an all women's race and the focus was on participation and not competition. The timing was perfect. I had been working on my doctorate for a number of years and had cut down drastically on my physical activity. I wanted to get back in shape and needed a goal.

When I signed up for the race, I wasn't exactly sure what the distances were, but I figured if I could swim for half an hour, run for half an hour, and ride my bike for an hour, I should be OK. It wasn't a very sophisticated approach to training but since I was already pretty active, it worked well for me. Best of all, it gave me a reason to prioritize my workouts and do them consistently. Swimming was the greatest challenge as I don't feel much of an inclination to jump into water unless it is 85 degrees and I am on a beach. But I figured that being rescued in the middle of the lake would not be a very auspicious beginning to my first triathlon and made myself go to the pool a day or two each week. I have a strong breaststroke; I just needed some confidence.

July came fast. As a first-timer, everything was exciting and inspiring and a little overwhelming. Running is an easy sport. You put on your shoes and you run. Getting organized for a triathlon is a bit of a production. But there was a great first-timers session at the bike drop-off the day before the race and the excitement was palpable. The triathlon itself was a blast. I wore my one-piece beach swimsuit (which I immediately recognized as a tactical error given the number of times I had to visit the porta-potty) and my pool goggles (which assured that I couldn't see a thing as the sun rose over the lake). But I was with supportive, enthusiastic women who were my age, I was not the sole breaststroker, and except for a brief moment of panic in the middle of the lake (when I realized I was in water over my head for the first time since I was a teenager), everything went fine.

At the conclusion of the swim, I staggered out of the lake, tried largely unsuccessfully to get dry socks on wet feet, had the strap on my bike helmet fall apart so it took me five minutes to get my helmet on, and then rode the entire bike ride in one gear (I used a borrowed bike which I had never learned how to shift). But riding my bike makes me feel like a kid again, and I realized as I rode (relieved that the swim was behind me) that at that point I had no expectations for myself except to have fun and finish. After years of self-imposed performance expectations (in running and almost every other area of my life), it was refreshing just to participate. I returned to the transition area without mishap, pulled my singlet with my race number on over my swimsuit, changed my helmet for my running hat, and took off... to the porta-potty, where I got to undo everything I had just done. So much for smooth transitions. The run, the portion I had pretty much taken for granted, turned out to be very challenging. (It finally occurred to me along the way that I didn't usually go for a swim and a bike ride prior to going for a run.) But as with every other leg of the race, the women around me continued to be encouraging and supportive.

The triathlon was an interesting experience for me because I was already an athlete, but I had not been in training for many years. Training again provided a wonderful discipline and rhythm to my life and helped me get back in touch with my physical self at a time when I was largely focused on intellectual pursuits. Best of all, it reminded me what it is like to take a risk and try something new. And finally, it was a humbling and inspiring experience to be surrounded by so many women with so many different stories which had brought them to that sandy starting line. Amidst the diversity of body types, abilities and challenges overcome was one common denominator—a positive attitude. That attitude celebrated the fact that whatever it had taken, we were all there together, and our youth and inexperience or our wrinkles and cellulite had nothing to do with the powerful women inside of us. And those were the women who completed this event. How could I not go back again and again?

Betsy Oudenhoven, a lifelong runner, has now completed three Danskin triathlons. This inspired her to buy a new bike and take swimming lessons. Betsy is married and the mother of two college students. After completing her PhD in November 2005, she took a position as the Vice President of Student Development at a community college.

FINISHING AND HAVING FUN
by Mary Beth Flanders

At the age of 43, I decided to retire from the rat-race that was the high-tech wireless telecommunications market. I'd been in the industry for twenty years and was frustrated with the pressures of international travel and the need to find balance in my life. My husband and I had three young children.

I decided to sign up for a triathlon; specifically, the Galena Triathlon in Northwest Illinois. It has a beautiful location, close to where my family has a second home, but the course is hard and hilly. I read that it was rated in the top 10 by USAT. The date was mid-May, and my biggest fear was that the swim would be cancelled if the water was too cold.

I had been working out for years, but wanted a radical change in results. I read that tri-sport training will put you in the best shape ever, and I decided that this change in focus was just what I needed. I had six months to train, and I devoted ten hours a week to the task. I was a member at a local Y and I found other triathletes to train with. My only goal was to finish the event and have fun. My husband and family agreed to support me at the race, but only if I didn't drag them into the training.

As race day approached I was prepared physically, but didn't feel I was getting enough time out in the open. Winter seemed to hang on forever, and on May first, I decided to completely move outdoors for the remainder of the training period. I had still not been in open water, and this had me a bit nervous. A friend offered to drive his boat alongside me while I swam at Lake Delavan. The water in the middle of the Lake was 53 degrees, and it was the first time I had swam in open water with a wetsuit. It was cold, but fun and exhilarating, and I decided I was ready.

I had been a lifeguard as a college student and was a runner for several years. I also had been on several century bike rides. All I needed was to put it all together in one morning. Seemed like no problem.

Two weeks before the race, I had a major setback. My husband was called to Brazil on business and wouldn't be able to get back for the race. He asked if I could find another support team. I was lucky that a good friend was planning on cheering on her sister for the race, and she took on that important job. She is a breast cancer survivor and she was quick to see how awesome her support would be. My sisters, my mom, and my niece also decided to join me for the day of the race, offering support along the route.

Everything went smoothly on the morning of the race. I was in the final wave of participants, and was with a small group of great over-40-year-old women. I swam without a problem, got on my bike, and took on the hills. Midway along the bike route, my family had stopped alongside the country road. I got off the bike for hugs and laughs. The policeman who was escorting me as the last rider asked if I wanted to quit. I declined his offer, but not the hugs of support. After 10 grueling miles, I met a woman whose bike was giving her trouble. She needed help with the chain, and I stopped to put it back on for her. I was bringing up the rear, and she was ready to quit. We decided to finish the ride together, and it was clear we both needed each other. She decided to bail out on the run, and after a quick transition, I headed out for the last event in the triathlon, the run.

I was the last woman across the finish line—since this wasn't a Danskin triathlon, there was a last woman!—but I wouldn't have changed a thing. Poi Dog Pondering's "Complicated" was playing as I crossed the finish line. I thought, "You bet, life is complicated, but it sure is fun." I had accomplished a great deal and met the goal I set: to finish the event and have fun. After the race, I felt incredibly good. I was full of energy, and wanted to party. My support team was exhausted at trying to chase me around all morning and deal with crowds. They shut me up with a couple of beers. Later I went on the Internet and printed out the results and realized that I spent way too much time in transition. This was my only big lesson—everything else was pure joy and fun.

Mary Beth Flanders is 46 years young! She's strong, crazy, and has a great deal of determination and energy. She loves her family, the mountains of Colorado, and all the free time that a furlough from corporate life has to offer. She had a hip replacement in 2005. Fully recovered, she returned to the sport of triathlon, including volunteering as a Workout Leader for the Chicagoland NW Suburbs Team Danskin Training.

When you set a goal, it's important that its meaning and purpose are consistent with what's most important to you. And here is a place where one's personal definition of success steps in. In addition to the significance of the goal itself, the way you achieve it will also express its meaning and purpose to you. Keep in mind that the meaning and purpose you seek will change.

Betsy's and Mary Beth's stories illustrate a challenge that so many of us face as women—trying to do it all. Given that we have a lifetime to achieve all our goals, the answer can be setting priorities and making the compromises that feel right for you at a certain point in life.

For Betsy, this meant putting athletic training on the back burner for a period of time while she worked on her PhD, maintained her career, and took care of family needs. It meant changing her athletic focus when she was ready to get fit again—trying something new like triathlon to overcome knees that just didn't work as well as they had in her younger years.

For Mary Beth, the answer was putting her career on furlough and embracing the challenge of doing a triathlon. Her new definition of success after leaving her work was to find more balance in her life. And her definition of success at that first triathlon was simply to finish and have a good time.

LESSON: Celebrate being in the game with your own definition of success.

Just as the very act of taking part in a triathlon is winning, simply becoming a more active participant in life is in itself winning too. Celebrate being alive!

If our focus is on perfectionism rather than the simple joy of participation, it's easy to get into a negative mind spiral of self-criticism, thinking about all the reasons why we are not "good enough." Life doesn't have to be that hard! Celebrate your strengths and forget your weaknesses. Do what you can in life, according to your own terms of success, and be glad for it.

WALKING WITH PRIDE
by Jennie Currie

Caught in a moment of weakness, I agreed to participate in the Orlando Danskin Triathlon last May with my mother and three sisters. This meant that I would have to EXERCISE! This is a word I seldom used—at least as it applied to me. My mother had been faithfully exercising since retirement; my sisters didn't have full-time jobs and so had time to exercise (at least that's what I always told myself). But I worked 10-11 hour days and didn't have time to sleep, eat, see my family (before bed), much less exercise!

I knew due to health reasons—I have fibromyalgia—I wouldn't have the energy to swim, bike AND run, but I could walk. My sister, Leah, arranged for two of her friends to join me as a relay team and the "1st Tri-ers" were born.

I was worried about finding the time to build up my strength and stamina enough to walk more than two miles. I knew if I didn't start walking immediately, it would take me hours to finish the triathlon. Fortunately, my co-workers came to the rescue. They suggested that I walk during lunch and if I didn't leave the building by 1 PM, someone would appear at my office door to "remind" me. Gradually, I worked up to 3 miles and knew I would be able to "pull my weight" during the triathlon itself.

I also knew that my fibromyalgia would make participating in the event difficult because the walking made me tired and was painful. Because I wanted to participate with my family, my doctor agreed to work with me and we came up with a plan to help me succeed without getting too tired or hurting too much. I crossed the finish line with my iPod and walking staff, feeling relaxed, comfortable, and proud!

I have so many people to thank for helping me accomplish something I didn't think possible: my husband and daughter, my doctor, co-workers and friends, sisters (and their friends), but most of all, my mom who made it all possible.

Thanks, Mom!

Jennie Curran, 48, along with Anne Sigler's three other daughters, participated in the Orlando Danskin together at Anne's insistence. (See related stories in Chapter 8.) Jennie, a Probation Officer, is from Houston, Texas. Married for 20 years, she has one daughter. Her interests include watching her daughter play volleyball and softball, reading, movies and visiting family.

Jennie's inspiring story is a perfect example of celebrating participation that is on your own terms.

For Jennie, getting to the start line was huge. Enjoying the journey was paramount. Finishing strong, as she defined it, given the circumstances of her life, was an accomplishment. Working toward and achieving her goal created confidence, courage, and an amazing sense of self-achievement.

Jennie's success involved more than the physical accomplishment of her walk. It also included completing an activity with her family—her mom and three sisters. Because they lived in geographically diverse locations, coming together was a cause for a celebration of family.

Jennie's experience illustrates a strategy of fulfilling multiple goals or needs in our lives by finding an activity that fulfills more than one need at once. Doing the Danskin with her family allowed Jennie to meet two needs at once—time with family and a way to get fit. An added advantage was that she was more likely to stick to her training schedule when she had triathlon partners to communicate with.

NOTE: Another way to combine multiple needs into one activity is by participating in an event that benefits a favorite cause. For example, many women are influenced to participate in the Danskin triathlon because a portion of the proceeds goes to breast cancer research.

LESSON: Learn from the journey, rather than focusing on the destination.

On one level, participating in a triathlon is about physical fitness and challenge… using a training plan and goal to improve your physical fitness. However, as we've observed, the training journey also provides other benefits and many life lessons.

What life journey are you on today? Why not look for the learning and benefits while you're "on your way"?

SHARING A NEW ADVENTURE
WITH AN OLD FRIEND
by Peggy Olson

The Danskin was an invitation to do something with a dear friend, a continuation down a road we've enjoyed for many years. Maybe I saw it as a reason to laugh or to add another memory to our treasure chest of friendship.

It was mid-April when the phone call came in. *"Hi Peg. What's up? How was Easter? How about doing a triathlon with me? The Danskin—swim, bike and run. It's short. We CAN do this."* Of course, my instant answer was, *"Us? Me? Are you nuts? No thanks!"*

I didn't consider myself an athlete but I am a person willing to give just about anything a try. So, with a little arm-twisting, I was in! July came, I was ready. We had recruited others to join us, but Sue and I stuck together.

We swam. I waited for her. We biked. She waited for me. We ran together. The finish line tied another knot in our already strong friendship.

What it's all about to me? A best friend to bring out the best in you. A shoulder, a hand, a push. Honesty with love. Laughing louder and longer.

Peggy Olson is the mother of three children, 20, 17 and 12 years old. She's been married 30 years. She did her first triathlon at 42 when her friend (the author) extended a challenge, knowing it would be accepted after the initial reservations, if for no other reason than to share a new adventure with a friend.

IT'S ALL ABOUT THE JOURNEY
by Dianne Michels

I am "doing the Danskin" for a variety of reasons. The number-one reason is probably the camaraderie and sense of magic that occurs when people join together in a common activity to achieve a shared goal.

I like that this goal is physical but it's also holistic in that it engages all of me relative to the training and the event itself—my mind, body, emotions and spirit.

It's exciting, challenging and rewarding to do something I've never done before and to have no idea about what will happen or how I'll feel.

The rigor and discipline required are appealing; a sense of being tested and rising to the occasion—like climbing a mountain or jumping out of an airplane—but this isn't as scary.

It's ironic, but the outcome seems less important to me than the journey of training and participating. The commitment is the accomplishment at some level because regardless of how well I do in the event, the gifts to my growth and development are in the training and the participation.

Wow!—I didn't know I felt this way about it. Thanks.

Dianne Michels is an HR and business consultant. These were her words as she prepared for her first triathlon (at the suggestion of the author) after relocating to Austin, Texas. She is the mother of two daughters, including Alison Garsson who also did the Austin triathlon, and has five grandchildren.

After the Danskin triathlons, some training teams have a post-celebration where the women ask themselves the following questions:

What did you learn?
What did this mean to you?

Taking the time to ask these questions is a form of celebration. It is a way of acknowledging what the women have gained, instead of simply moving on with less awareness.

Both Peggy's and Dianne's stories emphasize the experience and lessons of the journey to become a triathlete. Neither Peggy nor Dianne was especially concerned about finish times. They both possessed confidence that they would complete the goal they had set. What was most important to them was what they learned about themselves and their relationships along the way. It was about going outside of their comfort zones to try something new, and having a great time in the process.

LESSON: Don't set perfection as your standard. Allow yourself your humanity.

Those of us who are competitive and/or perfectionists by nature can be very hard on ourselves. When our focus is all about doing the best, every time, at everything we do, we may end up with unrealistic expectations that are impossible to attain. Then when we don't meet those expectations, we beat ourselves up and miss the positive aspects of all we've accomplished.

ALI'S REALIZATION
by author Susan L. Kane

I had the opportunity to sit down with Ali and her mom (Dianne Michels, whose story, "It's All About the Journey," appears above) to share our post-Danskin Austin observations. Ali, the mother of two young boys, was a classic overachiever. Having started out after college in New York City as an investment banker, she had a successful career before marrying, having two sons, and relocating to Austin. She recently had begun a career in real estate sales, at which her mother assured me would be a smashing success. In earlier years, Ali had completed a marathon or two.

After realizing her mother and one of her own friends were doing the Danskin, Ali decided to train for her first triathlon, too. Her schedule did not allow her to join the Team Danskin Training with her mom. So she hired a personal trainer, put together a plan, and then worked that plan. The night before the triathlon, Ali informed me that she intended to finish in less than an hour and 20 minutes, an ambitious goal for a first-timer. I figured that if Ali could do a marathon, she had a good chance of accomplishing her goal.

After the triathlon was over, Ali acknowledged that the swim was much harder than she expected. Her total time was about an hour and a half. But her next comment was the most interesting to me. Ali told me that after she had finished, she overheard a group of women discussing the out-of-town location for their next triathlon. Ali was astounded that these women who were WALKING the run (something that never would have been acceptable personally to Ali) were going to TRAVEL to do other triathlons. She then asked me, *Did I miss the point? Should I have tried to ENJOY the triathlon experience?*

Well, Ali, I thought, *there's no right or wrong answer. It's all about how you define success on your own terms.*

Alison Garsson, MBA, CFA, added the following to her story:
"As a follow on, I completed three more tris the following summer
and approached them as roughly a '90-minute workout'... not a
'race.' I had such a blast that I'm gearing up for more this season.
The best part is doing them with my girlfriends and not worrying
about my time."

BACK AGAIN!
by Susan L. Kane

One week after completing my fifth Danskin and five weeks
before my planned first co-ed international distance triathlon,
I woke up one morning with such excruciating pain. I could
barely get out of bed. Out of seemingly nowhere, I had a herniated disk in my back. It was a struggle to walk. Standing up in
the shower was an impossibility. Back surgery followed three
weeks later. Afterward, there was a lot of discomfort. Although
I had immediate relief from the pain that shot down the front
of my left leg to the knee, I had lost a lot of strength in that
leg. Three days after the back surgery, I went for my first walk.
It took me 30 minutes to walk a mile. What a contrast from
where I had been four weeks prior: in the best shape of my life,
almost ready to complete my first international distance tri!

Slowly, I regained strength and improved my walk times.
However, when I later tried to jog, it felt like there was a lead
weight attached to my left foot. *Step, slam, step, slam.* It took
three months of physical therapy to regain most of the strength
I had lost due to the nerve damage in my left leg.

The following summer brought a new triathlon season,
of course. I wondered whether I would be able to complete
another triathlon again. I decided to give my sixth Danskin
a try—my only goals being finishing and enjoying all the
positive energy of the day.

I trained and though I wasn't as strong and prepared as I had been the previous year, I felt ready for the race. Before the start of the triathlon, I made it a point to talk with women in my wave. I was inspired by the stories they told about why they were at the start line with me. In fact, I became so inspired that I later decided I needed to collect stories like theirs to include in a book (this one, of course!).

When I crossed the finish line that year, the experience was much like that of my very first triathlon. I cried tears of joy, feeling the rush of empowerment from my accomplishment. Once again, my health challenges did not prevent me from accomplishing this physical challenge. I had grown stronger and healthier through training.

Before that triathlon had started, I made a commitment to myself that I wasn't going to worry about my time. You see, the year before when I had done the triathlon feeling that I was in the best shape of my life, almost ready for the upcoming international distance tri, I had choked on the swim. Despite having done so much training, and becoming a better, stronger swimmer, I panicked. I made it through, but without the improvement I had expected on my swim time from prior years, without a sense of comfort in the water. I proceeded through the bike and run, still angry about my swim. And when I crossed the finish line that year, it was with tears of disappointment for not meeting my intended goals.

In the transition area, the year I was so angry, I passed a woman who told me it was one of the best days of her life! It hit me then. I would not do another triathlon unless I could be sure it was with a positive attitude. So, a year later, after recovering from back surgery, I decided I would just celebrate being there after all I had been through. I didn't care about my time—in fact, I wasn't even going to check my time.

A few days after that triathlon, however, my competitive spirit started to get the best of me. *You know, I think I really nailed the bike.* So I broke down and looked up my time. I couldn't believe it when I saw the results. After all I had been through with the effects of the back surgery, it took me a mere 1 minute and 13 seconds more than my time the prior year when I had felt so prepared. What a lesson I learned—focus on having a FUN, positive experience and the rest will fall into place. SHE WHO HAS THE MOST FUN WINS!

There's nothing like being around other women who are having fun to put perfectionist, harsh self-expectations into perspective. Beating yourself up while attempting a challenge is completely at odds with experiencing the joys of the journey and of self-discovery.

Alison set high expectations for herself in everything she did, including her first triathlon. The overachiever within her who had created a successful business career also drove her to set high goals for her triathlon endeavors. But demanding perfection kept her from enjoying the journey of the triathlon. How refreshing to see that Ali was able to set aside her high expectations and learn to have a "blast" while triing.

In getting to know Ali, I saw a lot of myself in her, although she is at least 10 years younger. However, she learned the lesson of enjoying the triathlon experience quicker than me. With each triathlon I trained for, I expected improvement over the time before. Anything less was not acceptable. When I didn't show the improvement I expected on the swim of my fifth triathlon, I took that as an opportunity to beat myself up, rather than congratulate myself for continuing to participate in triathlons while many of my friends no longer continued to tri.

When I put the emphasis on *celebrating* my participation in the triathlon after my back surgery, the self-imposed pressure of the past no longer existed. While focusing on having *fun*, I achieved results I could be proud of.

LESSON: Don't let age define what you can and can't do. Succeed on your own terms by staying healthy and vital.

Physical activity and fitness are the most important factors in successfully controlling the consequences of aging. Physical exercise and involvement in life trigger great waves of "grow" messages throughout the body and mind.

Fortunately, we have more information available to us nowadays about staying fit as the years add up. There's a way for you to stay in shape if you look for it, and the following two women found it in the Danskin triathlon.

JUDY'S START AT 66
by Judy Killion

I am a 66-year-old retired woman who never in a million years would have thought she would ever do *anything* athletic, let alone a triathlon. But I love to try new things to keep active and vital.

I decided to do my first triathlon at age 66 because my 30-something daughter asked me to join her in the Team Danskin Training where she would be a Workout Leader. There was a fair amount of "gray hair" in the class, but I think only one other lady in her sixties. We became friends and workout partners. Because I had previously trained to walk and completed a marathon, I firmly believed I could do the triathlon with training. And I felt that way right up until the day before the triathlon.

Saturday before "D" Day, we began with a breakfast potluck with our training teammates. Then we joined with the other Seattle area training classes for a "pep rally" with Sally Edwards. After that, we went to pick up our race packets and have our arms and legs marked. By then, I was a little nervous but was thinking, *It's okay.* My daughter and I met at the bike rack and I took a look around: where to go to swim, where to come back, where to exit and enter for biking, where the porta-potties were, etc. As I was driving home, I suddenly realized that there was no way I could do this. I was a terrible swimmer to begin with and, although I had taken two sets of swim classes and done many swim workouts, both in the pool and in the lake, I hadn't really improved. I wasn't afraid of drowning; I just knew it was going to take me a really long time and an awful lot of energy. I didn't think I'd have enough left for the biking and walking. I began to think that if I had a car accident on the way home, my classmates can't hold it against me when I chicken out.

But I made it home and curled up in my chair. Not too much later, my daughter and granddaughter arrived to spend the night since my daughter and I were going to go to the race together. I felt as if now I couldn't get out of it. I had a terrible night's sleep, waking up frequently and looking at the clock to see how much time I had left. Each time I awoke, I imagined myself getting into the water as soon as my wave was allowed on the ramp and kneeling down so that I would be wet up to my neck (I wouldn't be wearing a wet suit). We got up early, went through our last-minute checks of gear, water, food, etc., and took off.

Since I was in the second wave, I didn't have too much time to wait and stew. And when my wave got on the ramp, I went and got wet up to my neck just as I'd planned. And then I swam. And then I biked. And then I walked.

My daughter started about an hour and a half after I did, so she was able to see me into the water and out of it. She and my coach and assistant coach were there cheering me on as I stumbled out. My daughter helped me with my transition and then was off for her own swim. When I was about three-quarters of the way on the biking, she was coming the other way, saw me, and yelled, "Hi Mom!" I was so intent on not falling off my bike or getting in anyone's way that I didn't really see her, but yelled "hi" anyway. When I was about two-thirds of the way on the walking, she saw me and yelled, "Hi Mom!" After I had climbed the last hill and was a few blocks from the finish line, she caught up with me and we crossed the finish line hand-in-hand. What an incredible rush!

Now I'm going to do the Danskin until my granddaughter can join us. Then we'll be a three-generation Danskin family. My granddaughter is only four years old now so it's going to take a few years, but now I know I can do it. I may never do it any faster than I did this year, but I'll do it. And I may improve my time; I'll try to. But mostly, I'll do it. And I'm encouraging my peers to join me; they've known me for a long time. So they know they can do it if I can do it. We'll just keep adding to our circle and we'll all be healthier and the better for it. Hooray for the Danskin for encouraging women to do what they always thought they couldn't do.

Judy Killion is a 66-year-old retiree who volunteers where her heart leads her—ushering at theaters, making sandwiches for shelters, serving coffee and cookies to parents at a children's hospital, among other things. In additional to being a triathlete, she is a marathoner. Her daughter Gail Killion is a triathlete and Danskin WOL.

TRIATHLETE TRISH

She Who Has the Most Fun Wins!

If that's the standard, then it looks like I may be in contention for first place! I have enjoyed the training immensely. Muscles have sprouted where marshmallows used to live. My stroke is slow, my new bike is so fast it scares me, and my knees swell up when I try to jog. Still I am smiling all the time just thinking of how much fun this all is. Last year, I trained to walk a marathon. That was not nearly as much fun as the triathlon. The Danskin was sheer joy!

I am staring 60 in the eye and laughing!

Like Judy and Trish, let go of the assumption that you have to get *old*—that what you can and cannot do is determined by your age. Enjoy the wisdom and self-confidence that comes with maturity. At the same time, commit to staying physically active and remain engaged with life.

Consider Sally Edwards' experiences regarding aging and exercise. Sally was 33 when she completed her first Ironman Triathlon in 1980, finishing second among the women competitors with a time of 12 hours and 37 minutes. At 40, Sally set the record for the Masters level at the Ironman World Championship Triathlon. At 51, Sally came in second in the Women's Grand Masters category (50-and-over age class), losing by just 5 minutes to the winner. Sally's time of 10 hours and 42 minutes, at age 51, was the fastest Ironman of her life!

Sally's achievements demonstrate that age is not necessarily a hindrance in our physical accomplishments. One of Sally's motivations is to inspire others to redefine aging, to keep everyone—regardless of age—healthy and fit. She serves as a wonderful role model to many.

There's a wonderful message in these women's experiences… that is, to continue to enjoy life's journey and to keep adding new challenges. Be like Danskin triathlete Anne Sigler (Jennie Curran's mom from one of the previous stories), who not only decided to do her first triathlon at age 71, but insisted that all four of her daughters join the adventure!

Pacing Ourselves for a Fun Journey

As women, trying to have it all at once is not easy. In fact, it may be impossible without serious risks to your emotional health. The good news is that you CAN do it all—family, career, physical fitness, hobbies, passions, giving back—just maybe not all at once.

Earlier it was mentioned that we have a lifetime to achieve all our goals. So to keep the fun in your approach to life, it can be helpful to think of *sequencing* the things you want to accomplish. Sequencing is about looking at what makes sense to prioritize in your life right now.

Maybe this is the period in which you want to make the most time for school, your job, your family? What makes the most sense for you now, and will keep you smiling? How can you add physical activity into the mix? Is it the perfect time to get involved in a triathlon? Or do you want to save that for another phase? Or is some other physical activity more in line with what will work for you at this point?

Pacing ourselves keeps the fun in our living, in our doing, and in our being.

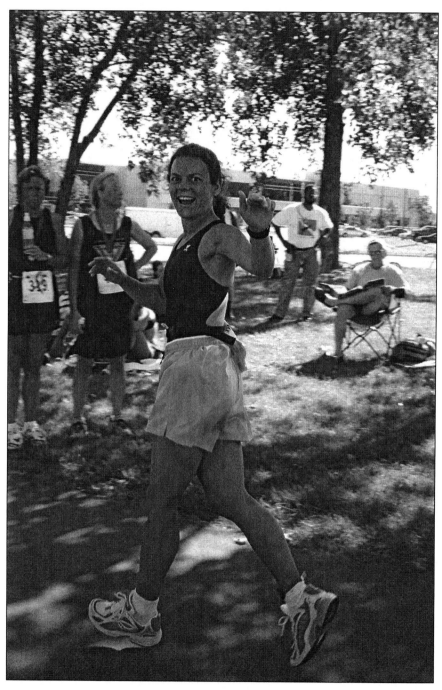

TRIATHLETE JENNIFER BURKE

CHAPTER 4

Follow Your Passion

> *"What is triathlon?*
> *It's exercise. It's fitness. It's being healthy.*
> *It's a way of life. It's my passion.*
> *Triathlon has given me unbelievable confidence*
> *that transcends the race course.*
> *I always thought I could do anything I wanted to,*
> *but now I actually believe it!"*
> – Susan Farago

Think of a time when you noticed someone who was obviously enthusiastic and passionate about their life—someone who had that special spark. Didn't you want to have that spark, too? Or maybe you *are* that sparkling person some of the time—do you long to be in that space more often?

In her book, *In My Wildest Dreams*, author Gail Blanke encourages us to identify what brings us great joy. Besides experiencing greater enjoyment ourselves, she points to an additional bonus. When we're moving in the direction of our passion, we become that person with a special spark who inspires others to live their dreams.

Today women are discovering or re-discovering the experience of feeling passionate—of feeling truly alive, energetic and in "the Zone"—through becoming involved in the challenge of a triathlon.

LESSON: In taking care of yourself, you may discover a passion!

In Chapter 2, we discussed the need to take care of *you*. By including self-care as one of your top priorities, you'll become a happier, more energetic person. Optimally, if you can live a life that is fueled by your passion, you will have boundless energy. Work will no longer seem like work. Time will fly by as you put your efforts into activities that you love. Others will be attracted to your energy and derive energy from you.

Both of the following stories illustrate what happens when a woman begins taking care of herself, and in the process, discovers a passion for the triathlon.

TRI THIS FOR HALF-TIME ENTERTAINMENT!
by Sarah Berszoner

I am at what is, I like to think, the midpoint in my life (53, as viewed by USAT standards). I finally have the opportunity to enjoy the half-time entertainment, which I hope to extend for a least three more decades. I saw a saying, "Life is a Tri, Go for It!" and that's my plan for the future.

When I was in my late forties, I decided I wanted to be "Fit at 50." My husband was seriously ill with several major medical issues at the time. We spent a good part of the last five years in and out of medical facilities. Throughout this period in my life, I was a caregiver at home while working "full-time plus" in the corporate world. Needless to say, this was a somewhat stressful lifestyle. I decided to do everything possible to improve my health because, while some health issues cannot be avoided, many can be eliminated with positive lifestyle choices.

I started working with a personal trainer toward my new fitness goal. The focus was primarily strength training, using

cardio activities as a warm-up, and while the routine was effective for weight loss and general conditioning, building aerobic capacity was missing. I've always enjoyed various sports,
am reasonably coordinated, and liked being active, but never
really found my niche. I've secretly wanted to be a competitive athlete in some sport and was excited when the magazine
GeezerJock was first published because it provided examples
of successful athletes in every sport imaginable over the age
of 40.

I worked with two people on an extensive project at work,
one an accomplished triathlete who was mentoring the other
as a newbie. I was fascinated by the sport and impressed that
these two got up at 4 AM to swim and train before a hectic day
in the world of public accounting. As I tweaked my fitness pro-
file, I was seeking something that not only would be challenging, but also could be done throughout life. Triathlons seem
like the perfect choice, because you don't just run—which can
be really tough on older joints—rather you mix it up and swim
and bike, too. You also incorporate weight-bearing exercises
and core work, which ward off osteoporosis for older women
like me; so it's the perfect recipe for the "Baby Boomer" crowd.
I talked to my work triathlete friend about giving it a "tri" and
she agreed it was perfect for someone my age. She assured me
that I, too, could be a triathlete, but highly recommended formal training with someone experienced in the sport.

I decided to attempt a sprint distance triathlon just to
see if I could cross the finish line intact. I registered for the
Chicagoland Danskin. Having told family and friends my
plan, I was now committed and knew I had to start training
for the event. I took a triathlon group class during the winter/
early spring at my health club, which was a great introduction to the sport. The group class was fun and I learned a lot,
ranging from swimming technique to changing a bike tire.
However, I didn't think I was disciplined enough to train the

way I should on my own. So I joined Team Danskin Training after my health club class ended, with a wonderful group of women in the northwest suburbs of Chicago.

Coach Susan Kane was exceptional in charting out the training course and ensuring that we had as much information as possible. Coach Susan and Coach Jean Spiegelhalter were both extremely knowledgeable about the three disciplines with the added bonus of having triathlon event experience. They, along with the other Workout Leaders, were always encouraging and urged us to work outside our comfort zone for improvement, but they were always considerate of our conditioning levels. The heart rate-monitoring instruction was invaluable and was always coordinated with every activity. It was awesome truly feeling that you were part of a team, even though we all had varying ability levels.

July arrived and it was D-Day for the Danskin. We met as a team on Saturday. We were briefed on details a novice would never even think about on her own; it was great. Sally Edwards spoke to our team, which was really special and quite inspiring. I made it through the Danskin with 3,900 other women and finished, which was my goal. I had a great time because my focus was fun, not speed. After this crossing the finish line of my first triathlon, I was very motivated to improve, having awakened my competitive spirit, coupled with my desire for fitness for life. I became truly passionate about the sport. It made me want to be a better all-around person in all aspects of my life. Life is indeed a journey with twists and turns along the way; however, I feel that for all the doors which have been closed (my husband passed away the prior January), my Danskin training group and the event itself opened a double-door of opportunity for my future.

I had a feeling triathlons would be the thing for me. I participated in another sprint distance tri in August for more race experience and to see if I really liked the sport. The answer was a resounding "yes!" Triathlons are challenging and fun and involve a great community of people. I should be able to train for triathlons for the long term. I'm now serious about this and have hired a coach to improve all of my tri skills so I can advance further in the sport. I like that it's an individual effort (except for the coaching aspect and the events themselves) and you're really only competing with yourself. There's a saying that "the more you know, the more you realize how little you know." I've only scratched the tri surface, but am looking forward to learning for a long time. I'm extremely grateful for the wonderful Danskin experience that has been life-changing. I've discovered a true passion!

Sarah Berszoner lives in Bolingbrook, Illinois. She is the mother of a son, who graduated from the United States Air Force Academy in the midst of training for her first triathlon.

DO MORE, DO IT BETTER
by Jennifer Burke

The Danskin race in Pleasant Prairie, Wisconsin began what is now my passion for the sport. I know I will be involved for the rest of my life at any age as a participant, volunteer or spectator.

I started out with a simple desire to get back in shape after the birth of my second daughter. My body was definitely not the same and could not take the constant pounding of running. Also, I had what I refer to as my "mini-mid-life crisis." I was overwhelmed! How could I do it all and do it all well? Wife, mom, breadwinner, employee, community, personal health? YIKES! Danskin helped me get a grip on my life and prioritize the important stuff. As a side bonus, I also got into the best shape of my life.

I continued to do other sprint distance triathlons. After the birth of my third daughter, I set my sights on the Chicago Accenture race. I was greatly inspired by the incredible athletes around me and wanted to do more and do it better. I enjoyed the adrenaline rush. My days of getting that rush by parachuting out of planes and bungee-jumping off cranes were over—I needed something more constructive in their place.

I've learned a lot about myself from this passion for the sport. When I'm well-balanced, I am a better mom, wife, boss and friend. And I'm having a lot more FUN! There's no limit to what you can accomplish. It's just what you choose to accomplish and WHEN you choose to accomplish it. It's all about priorities. Don't ever give up. Always strive to better yourself.

I even inspired my husband to get into the sport. (*If SHE can do it, I certainly can.*) He's now training for an Ironman. I could never do any of this without his full support, especially on my training and race days. Fortunately, we share the same passion for triathlon, which is a neat bond to have. Maybe someday our daughters will be inspired to join us!

Jennifer Burke, 39, is a wife, as well as the mother of three daughters (Emma, 9; Sarah, 6; and Katie, 3). She works full-time as a VP of Sales for a marketing services company. Jennifer lives in Glen Ellyn, Illinois.

Mihaly Csikszentmihalyi, author of the classic book, *Flow*, notes that the best moments of our lives come when a person's body or mind is stretched to its limit in a voluntary effort to accomplish something difficult and worthwhile. "Optimal experience" is described as a time when we "feel in control of our actions, masters of our own fate." Both Sarah and Jennifer created this passionate optimal experience through the triathlon and other athletic goals, interests originally generated by a wish to take better care of themselves.

As part of her self-care, Sarah decided to make fitness a priority. This decision came as she watched her husband's health deteriorate. Even though Sarah worked a demanding full-time job and was her husband's primary caregiver, she made the time to work out. Sarah set the goal to be "Fit at 50." She continued to search for activities and goals that would be motivating to her. Shortly after her husband's death, Sarah committed to working with a triathlon training group at her health club. Over the next several months, Sarah discovered that she had a passion for triathlon—which she views as a long-term solution for keeping herself healthy and motivated.

Meanwhile, Jennifer's challenges were typical of the challenges many women face today—trying to balance family, career, community and personal health. What began as a way to do something for herself—training for her first Danskin to get back in shape after having her second daughter—eventually turned into a passion that both Jennifer and her husband could share. She found joy and satisfaction in competing in triathlons, upping the ante to participate in the Chicago Accenture triathlon. Like Sarah, she expects triathlon, in one form or another, to be always be a part of her life.

LESSON: Once you find it, passion easily becomes the center of your life.

Passion is a critical component of success. Passion provides fuel to transform work and other activity into joy, into moments of "flow" where you are so absorbed in what you are doing that you lose track of time.

A spark of passion was ignited in the following two women through triathlon. With passion as the center, participating in triathlons became a lifestyle that brings joy amidst all their other responsibilities in life.

FINDING THE PASSION WITHIN
by Amanda Betlow

My first tri… then my second… and then… on to Kona?

Why did I decide to train for my first triathlon? At the suggestion of my friend, Sara, to try something different. Little did I know how my life was about to change!

My adventure began on a cool March morning eight weeks prior to the May Danskin race which was to be held on the Disney properties in Orlando, Florida. I attended my first Multisport Co. training group practice. Lea Murdoch and Lori Croft were the two head coaches while other ladies were introduced as team leaders. Having come from an athletic background, I thought that the training would be a cinch. Boy, was I WRONG! The first bike practice left me discouraged because I was so slow, but I was determined to improve. During my first swim workout, I thought the lady in the lane next to me, treading water, was moving faster than I was swimming. At least I was happy with my running ability from the start!

Over the weeks, my swimming improved. I became a fish in the water and the swim became my strongest leg of the race. Lea and Laurie kept pushing me on my bike rides to get faster and more comfortable prior to race day. Finally, the bike and run brick workouts prepared me for the switch during the race and feelings of transitioning from one sport to the other. After eight weeks, I was amazed with the progress I made. I was hooked before I even crossed the finish line of my first Danskin race. I signed up for the Olympic distance triathlon which was also to be held at Disneyland in Orlando in September.

One of the mottos for the Danskin Triathlons is "When is the last time you did something for the first time?" Competing in the Danskin marked the last time I did a triathlon for the first time because, when I crossed that finish line, I became a triathlete!

Four days after the Danskin race, I fell off my bike and fractured two bones in my elbow. I lost six weeks of training time for my weakest link because of that setback. I knew I would have to get back on the bike, overcome the fear that came from my fall, and ride like never before. When I was able to ride again, I was more determined than ever.

I was hooked, but anxious about the September Olympic distance triathlon. I signed up for more guidance through Lea's and Laurie's summer/fall race training program. I loved the team interaction as well as individual training. I thought it would be a good idea to get another race under my belt prior to the September race so I signed up for the Moss Park Sprint on July 15th. The distance was longer than the Danskin, and I felt a bit intimidated. However, with the great training techniques from my two terrific coaches and the support of other friends (Kathy, Tamar and Sara), I knew there would be no stopping me. I felt a lot more confident in myself than I did prior to the Danskin race.

Upon finishing, I saw my time was 1:34—only four minutes off from my planned race time. I was happy; I packed up my belongings and left the race with my head held high. Little did I know until I got the official results from the race that I had placed second in my age group! A new goal emerged as I became more passionate about the sport: I would perfect my bike for the September race.

Overall, my triathlon experiences have been positive and uplifting. An inspiring quote I found along the way was, "Passion is finding potential within and having the power to unleash it." I have discovered abilities I never knew I had. I am looking to further my triathlon races and increase distances over the years and race an Ironman. I have hopes and dreams of Kona. I've learned the only one stopping me from achieving anything is me. By pushing myself a little more each time and unleashing the power of passion within me, I know I will be able to achieve my dreams and goals—though always with the help of great friends and my supportive family.

As planned, Amanda Betlow completed her first Olympic distance triathlon, on a day that was only one month after her step-father passed away suddenly. In addition to her own training goals, Amanda has exhibited her passion for triathlon by becoming an Orlando Team Danskin Training Workout Leader. She has since completed her first half-Ironman distance race.

FROM DANSKIN TO IRONMAN HAWAII
by Susan Farago

How could I ever have known the impact the Danskin Women's Triathlon would have on my life when I turned 30 in 2000? It would challenge my physical abilities, my mental fortitude, and my beliefs about who I am and what I am capable of. I had no idea what the years since then would bring!

When I turned 30, I was working long hours for a company that cared less about me than I did of it. In my attempt to get back in shape, I took up running when I was 28. By my 30th birthday, my knees were starting to protest from all the pounding they had endured over the past two years. I came across a flyer at the local running store that advertised the Danskin Women's Triathlon. I discovered from the flyer that a triathlon was swimming, biking, and running. I figured I already knew how to swim, I could run (despite what my knees told me), and I had a mountain bike I could use. Feeling the need to try something different, I went online and signed up for the race. I told my husband, Leary, about it the next day. "You're doing a WHAT?!" was his response. I had two months to get ready.

The first thing I did was get out a calendar and start writing in the days I would "train." I knew nothing about bricks (bike/run combinations), I thought "periodization" referred to what "came once a month," and really didn't understand the difference between swimming in open water and in a pool. Nutrition was something related to the food pyramid and carbohydrates were viewed as "evil" according to Dr. Atkins. In my usual approach to things, I knew where I wanted to go but didn't know how to exactly get there. Ignorance was bliss! So after about 30 minutes of penciling workouts on a calendar, I had my plan. I referred to that calendar nearly every day for those two months. The only training buddy I had was Leary, who would ride his mountain bike alongside me when I ran (to make sure nothing happened to me), or would come find me in his truck as I rode my mountain bike around town (to bring me food and, again, to make sure nothing happened to me). I was a better swimmer than Leary was so he left me on my own in the pool, probably figuring that if anything did happen to me I could just stand up.

Race day came, and Leary and I made our way out to the race site. Neither one of us really knew what to expect. I got my equipment area set up (I didn't know it was called a "transition") and waited for the race to start. It started to rain but that didn't bother me—I was just so excited! I had no idea what the day would bring but I was ready for it. There were so many women racing—nearly 2,000! I felt like I was at some type of National Organization for Women convention—except that most of us were in our bathing suits. I knew the race would go fast, like some type of time warp, so I made a point to look around and be in the moment. I remember certain parts of that morning like they were yesterday. I remember the feeling of getting into the cool lake water with all the other women in my age group and thinking how very weird it would be swimming with everyone. But once the gun went off, it was exhilarating to be in the open water. Seventeen minutes later, I finished the swim. Time seemed to fly by as I ran up the AstroTurf path to where the bikes were racked. I had on a two-piece bathing suit and I remembered thinking that I should probably NOT be running given the lack of support in my suit. But there were so many people lining the runway up to the bikes that I just HAD to run! (I would later get my race photos back and my fears were confirmed—NEVER run in a two-piece bathing suit while wearing a swim cap. It is not attractive and gravity exaggerates EVERYTHING!!)

I took my time in transition to change clothes—why hurry? The notion of "fast transitions" was completely unknown to me. Nearly 7 minutes later, I emerged from transition wearing dry clothes, helmet, fashion sunglasses with pink tinted lenses, and I had my trusty 50-pound mountain bike. The bike course was hilly but there was only one hill I was really worried about and it was near the end of the ride. I tried not to think about it. Instead, I focused on the beautiful park scenery and making my way around all the women who had flat tires on their super speedy road bikes. Not so speedy now! Good thing I had my big nubby mountain bike tires! The big hill finally came and my goal was to get to the top without getting off my bike. There were plenty of women walking their bikes up the hill but not me. I was breathing so hard I thought my heart was going to explode in my neck! But I kept turning the pedals over slowly, thanked no one in particular for my triple chain ring, and as I crested the top of the hill, I smiled and yelled, "YEAH! I MADE IT!" Shortly thereafter, I made my way back into the park area and followed the spectator-lined street into transition. There was Leary cheering me on louder than anyone else. It was great to see him and it gave me a boost of confidence. Forty minutes from when I started the bike, I was already done. Once in transition, all I had to do was drop off my bike and helmet and pick up my running hat and water bottle holder, since I wore my running shoes on the bike ride. This would explain why I only spent three minutes in transition this time around. I made my way out onto the run course. It was so humid but thankfully, it was also still cloudy. I ran out of the park area and I had to be careful with my footing as some of the trail areas had since turned into mud. Once out onto the paved road, I ran and ran and ran. It was great! I had no idea how fast I was running but it was just amazing to be out there with all these other women, spectators cheering us and us cheering each other.

As I ran back into the park, I knew this was going to be over very soon and I didn't want it to end. I came back into the park and could hear the announcer at the finish line. I ran around the corner and down towards transition. I saw Leary again, yelling and cheering me on. I couldn't believe I was about to finish the race! I crossed the finish line just as the announcer said my name and when I stopped running, a volunteer put a finisher's medal around my neck. I heard someone yelling my name and I turned around and saw Leary. I ran right into his arms. "You did it! You did it!" he kept saying over and over. He was grinning just as big as I was and he hugged me and picked me up into the air. I finished in 1 hour, 36 minutes. I had no idea if this was fast or slow. I didn't care. I finished!!!!!!! I held up the medal to Leary and said, "You know what? I HAVE to do another one of these things!" And so I did.

In the six years following that first race, I am still doing "these things." I have come to love and embrace triathlon as a lifestyle—a lifestyle I share with my husband who is now also a triathlete. My persistent thirst for more, more, more and farther, farther, farther has led me to complete all race distances: sprint, Olympic, half-Ironman, and Ironman. It took me nearly four years to work my way up (mentally and physically) to the idea of doing a full Ironman. After all, that distance is only for crazy people! But I have come to realize that "going long" is my favorite distance, and between 2004 and 2006, I completed four Ironman races, including qualifying for and participating in the Ironman World Championship in Hawaii in 2005.

I never thought I would be talking about the Danskin Women's Triathlon and Ironman Hawaii as they are as far apart as day and night. One is not better than the other; they are just two different animals—but both animals nonetheless. Without Danskin, I would have never made it to the Ironman World Championships in 2005. Danskin introduced me to the sport, and after five years of hard work and dedication, I found myself amongst the greatest triathletes in the world. I felt like such a poser. While Leary and I were in Kona, people would come up to us, turn to Leary and say, "So are you excited about the race?" He would correct them and proudly declare that it was me, not him, doing the race. We were met with this type of sexist assumptions quite frequently and it came from the spectators and locals, not from the athletes. The athletes knew better. Kona was an amazing experience and racing through the lava fields with professional triathletes and top age groupers alike was an experience I will never forget. But it was Danskin that gave me my first taste of this sport and to this day, I hold my Danskin finisher's medal on par with my Ironman Hawaii medal.

When I participated in Ironman Wisconsin in September 2006, the race statistics showed only 25% of participating athletes were women. This statistic had not changed at all from 2004 when I did that same race. Yet for many of the shorter distance races, average race statistics show 50% or more of participating athletes are women. Why? Is it simply lack of desire for women to push ourselves farther or harder? Or is it more likely a reflection of the times where women have more responsibilities than their counterparts and are still unable or unwilling to take time for themselves?

Triathlon is a lifestyle. I didn't understand this until I became a triathlete. And I didn't consider myself a triathlete for several years. But now, I live to swim, bike, and run. And these activities aren't things I have to do, they are not extras, and they don't get in the way of my job or my family. But rather they are integrated into everyday activities just like wiping off countertops, getting dressed, or putting gas in the car. It is not only about the actual sports but what those sports have come to represent. They represent long Saturday-morning bike rides with friends—which can turn into afternoon bike rides when training for an Ironman. They represent Sunday-morning runs around Townlake with friends, followed by a cold leg soak in Barton Springs, and then pancakes or breakfast tacos afterwards. They also represent learning what to eat and what not to eat, traveling to race venues, sharing injury complaints and massage therapist recommendations, and getting rid of the dining-room table to make way for the treadmill and bike trainer. And beyond that, these three sports have enabled friends to become good friends through long runs and deep conversations about jobs, relationships, and the meaning of life.

What is triathlon? It's exercise. It's fitness. It's being healthy. It's a way of life. It's my passion. Triathlon has given me unbelievable confidence that transcends the race course. I always thought I could do anything I wanted to, but now I actually believe it!

Susan Farago is supported by her wonderful husband Leary, who is also a triathlete, and her cat Fritz, who is not. She is an active member of Austin Triathletes. When Susan is not running, swimming, biking, eating or sleeping, she works full-time as a project manager at IBM and enjoys writing and gardening.

Let's face it… you have to be pretty passionate about triathlon in order to want to do an Ironman triathlon, which involves a 2.4-mile swim, a 112-mile bike ride, and a 26-mile run (the length of a typical marathon). Through a Danskin sprint-distance triathlon, a passion was discovered that was previously unknown for Amanda and Susan. After identifying the need for a challenge, the watershed was open as each found an opportunity to use their skills and abilities.

For these two women, training—which those without passion for triathlon would consider "work"—was joyful. It provided an opportunity to share time with friends and realize new adventures. Although training was physically demanding, it probably appeared effortless to others. Because of their natural abilities and love for athletic pursuits, Susan and Amanda were able to train longer and harder.

LESSON: Love what you do and know that it matters.

Many of you reading this book share a passion for triathlons. Yet what motivates and drives one reader in other areas of her life may be completely different from the next reader. One person may also be passionate about painting, another for mountain climbing, still another toward working soup kitchens. The important thing is to find what gets *you* jazzed.

In finding what fuels your passion, you'll develop a clear vision of where you want to go, a sense of purpose. You'll know that you're doing what you love, using your unique skills and talents, and accomplishing what's important to you. The world benefits because your actions serve others.

In the next story, triathlon leads a woman to making many positive changes and discovering a passion beyond her own participation in the sport.

DISCOVERING MY PASSION HAS BEEN MY BLESSING
by Sharon Spencer

I am one of those women who has struggled with my weight all my life. After having three children and gaining 50 extra pounds, I found myself depressed and rather alone. I was emotionally at my lowest. Having struggled for years through the military and college with an eating disorder, I knew it could easily return and I had to do something.

I did a lot of praying and soul-searching and found my focus to be completing the Danskin race. I had actually signed up for the two previous years' races and backed out because I didn't think myself worthy of such an event. I began a regular exercise program and developed a new attitude about food. I started to see results. I focused on fitness instead of dieting and regularly visited the Danskin site for encouragement and tips. I read Sally Edwards' book, *Triathlons for Women*, and finally began to see myself as belonging. In short, 55 pounds of weight loss later, and three seasons full of triathlons including two Danskin races and a half-iron aquabike, I am a new person. My friends and family are amazed at the transformation and I give so much credit to Danskin for what they offer to so many women.

This past summer, I coached three girlfriends for the Chicagoland race and, wow, do we have a story to tell! After dragging my girlfriend out of her own puke on the swim, I spent 20 minutes in transition trying to prepare my girlfriends for the bike. We pulled out on the course only to find the Team Danskin "sweep team" and the truck with the light pulling up the rear behind us. In other words, we were at the very back of the pack. I tried not to let my friends know that and just focused on the road ahead, but they were soon aware of where we were in the race. Lauren Jensen, a professional triathlete who was part of the sweep team (and had placed first in the race), was simply amazing in her support of my friends and her manner of encouragement. She was quite honestly a true blessing from above for them, never once mentioning she actually was a pro. As we entered transition for the second time, a crew of Team Danskin runners was waiting with encouragement and support. They stuck with us through the run and we finished in a blaze of glory together (and not last!).

I found a true passion in leading my friends through the race and not just "going for it" on my own. I am working toward leading an even larger group of women to at least the Chicagoland race, if not another as well. But I would like to find a way to do even more. Danskin has touched my life in such a way that I feel compelled to do more, and to show other women what we can accomplish together. Throughout many of my other races, there are moments where I, as an athlete, felt every much alone and on my own. Danskin is completely different, and brings out an even greater success than any other race. It is women as a whole, working together toward a victory of completion, toward finding and grasping that magical something that empowers you to do anything.

I want to find a way to turn my passion for this sport, for women's fitness, for Danskin, into something more. I will be completing the Level 1 triathlon coaching certification through USAT this off-season, as well as training myself for an Ironman-distance race. I am looking for ways to share my passion with other women, whether it be through coaching, training, or motivating. I look forward to a continued dedication and devotion to Danskin in return for the life-changing gift I have received!

Sharon Spencer is a wife as well as a mother of three children, ages 11, 9 and 4, in Oxford, Michigan. As a result of her Danskin experiences, she has joined a cycle racing team and is training for a half Ironman and full marathon in the upcoming season. She is studying to become an ACSM certified personal trainer.

Training for her first triathlon brought many benefits to Sharon. She lost weight, got physically fit, and overcame depression and an eating disorder. As a result of her self-described "transformation," fitness is now an important part of Sharon's daily life. However, she found her true passion combined the newfound physical and emotional fitness with helping others.

In coaching women for their first Danskin races, Sharon found that she was using her unique talents and gifts to help others, which really got her excited. She created her own energy and spread the energy and excitement to others. This passion provided clarity of purpose. As a result, she decided to further develop her coaching skills through USAT and Team Danskin Training. Her enthusiasm and passion are contagious and help to make the world a better place.

Find Your Passion and Make It Happen!

For each of the stories in this chapter, passion for triathlons or coaching was unleashed by "being out there," by trying something new. To make this possible, the women had to make room in their lives to explore a new interest. And as their interest grew into a passion, they gave it a high priority in their life.

If you haven't already made your passion a key part of your life, it's essential that you do so now. This is how we create a joy-filled life.

You may not start out knowing what your passions include. Given a chance, maybe you'll discover that athletics is a part of this. Or perhaps you've already reconnected with your ability to feel passionate through the Danskin Triathlon or other athletic goals.

Take time now to also consider other ways that you might tap into your passion. What excites you? What brings you great joy? What is something new you'd like to explore? Know that by using personal strengths that bring you joy, you'll be best able to discover and realize your life's purpose. And by identifying your passions—for your personal time *and* at the office—and creating a life that honors those passions, you'll readily create connections and community with others.

Sally Edwards provides a wonderful example of someone who has found her life purpose based on her passions. Sally's current passions include getting Americans fit and empowering women. Her strengths include being a natural athlete (which drove her activities in earlier years) and being an inspirational and motivational speaker. Through her activities as the National Spokewoman of the Danskin Triathlon Series, founder of Heart Zones USA and The Sally Edwards Company, and as a public speaker and author, Sally has motivated thousands to make fitness the cornerstone of their lives. Sally inspires others to work harder and longer than they thought possible. Anyone who has been around Sally can't help but be impressed by her seemingly endless energy and obvious passion for what she does. As illustrated by many of the stories in this book, Sally's energy and passion are contagious and inspiring.

Investigate YOUR passions, as they relate to your life purpose and otherwise. Then *set goals* related to your passions, which will be discussed further in the next chapter.

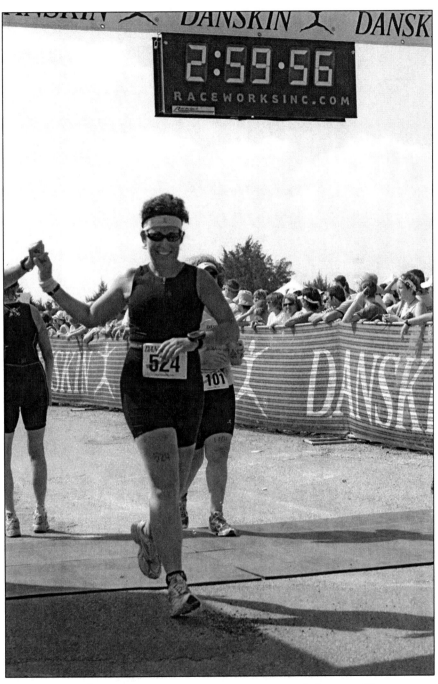

SUSAN KANE AT THE FINISH LINE OF THE 2006 AUSTIN DANSKIN
(PHOTO COURTESY OF BRIGHTROOM.COM)

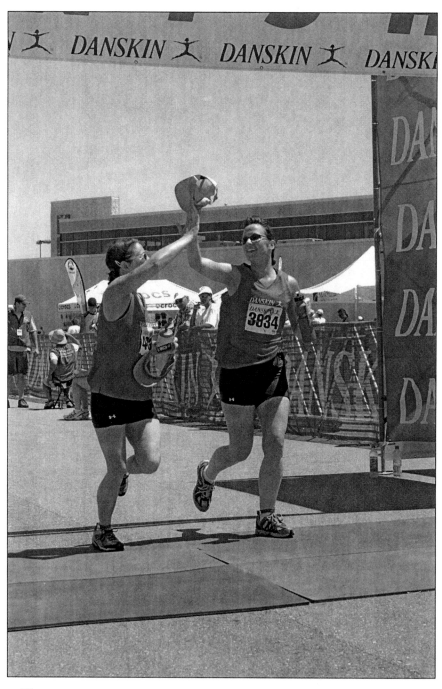

TRIATHLETES ACHIEVE THEIR GOAL OF CROSSING THE FINISH LINE.
(PHOTO COURTESY OF BRIGHTROOM.COM)

Chapter 5

The Value of Goals and Challenges

> *"When was the last time you did something for the first time?"*
> – Danskin slogan

Setting a goal for yourself is necessary for achievement. Goals focus our energy, reduce distractions, and give meaning to our desires. In turn, it is your desires, values and beliefs that cause you to set the goal and take action in the first place.

According to Brian Tracy, the author of *Maximum Achievement*, human beings are goal-centered, motivated by purposes and desired end-states. We are never really happy until and unless we are moving toward the accomplishment of something that is important to us. "When you are excited about achieving a clear major goal, you start to move forward rapidly in spite of all obstacles and limitations," he tells us.

The likelihood of achieving your goal is highest if it is *challenging, but doable*. According to Tracy, it should have at least a 50% or better probability of success.

LESSON: Having a *well-defined, measurable goal* provides motivation.

You can't read one of Sally Edwards' books on fitness without reading about the value of goals. Sally Edwards believes that: "every fitness program requires goals." She recommends establishing specific smaller goals that can help you mark your progress and keep you motivated for your larger overall goal.

Is your major goal fitness-related or associated with some other aspect of life? In either case, you'll find that it's the setting of well-defined and measurable smaller goals that will keep you energized and on track.

WITH A GOAL, I GOT OFF THE COUCH
by Laurel Collins

It's amazing how easy it is for me to blow off exercise if I don't have a concrete goal. I was kind of dragged into doing my first Danskin. When I was first approached by my personal trainer, Niki, I said, "No way," even though we had been working together for almost a year. After being talked into joining Team Danskin Training though, I found it really made me find the time, energy, and child care to bike, run, etc., as scheduled. It was great having a training schedule. When I had tried to work out on my own in the past, when Niki wasn't around, there was always some chore that needed to get done and that mighty comfy couch. It was amazing how committed I was to training for my goal, the NY Metro Danskin. I always found a way to get it done.

Prior to starting to work out with Niki, I hadn't been physically active in years, but it wasn't that I was never active in the past. I had been involved in gymnastics and dance since childhood. In high school, I ran track and cross country. I even learned to ice skate as an adult, and my husband and I used to mountain bike—but all that was over 13 years ago before I had my kids.

In terms of body image, like many women, I was struggling with those last 10 pounds. (Hey, my whole life, I was a size four until I had kids.) I told myself that if I didn't lose any weight after working out four or five days a week, then 137 was just my post-pregnancy weight and that was that.

The day of the race was great. I knew my swim would be very slow. Five waves of women got into the water, swam past me, and got out before I finished! But I did what I could do, and even though I had to walk most of the 5k due to leg cramps, it was exhilarating to cross the finish line with a woman I met on the run, Eileis Andreas. We had so much in common, and in those few minutes, we really bonded and crossed the finish line holding hands!

Training for the triathlon to reach my goal is what pushed me from being a couch potato at heart to the athlete I used to be. I feel like myself again. I always complained about having to exercise, hating it, though I knew it was a necessary evil. I've turned the corner and now, with goals in hand, actually like challenging myself. I have not lost one blessed pound, but I have gained tremendous amounts of self-esteem and positive body image. Instead of looking in the mirror and seeing the post-baby pooch on my belly, I see an athlete.

Laurel Collins, 38, is the mother of two boys, ages 6 and 8. She completed the NY Metro Danskin (Sandy Hook) triathlon in 2006.

MY GOAL, MY GIFT
by Cyndi Sunby

I had always been somewhat active through my 20s and 30s doing dance classes, aerobic tapes, snow skiing, etc. Even into my 40s, I would generally have a good routine for 8 to 10 months, but then would slide into inactivity for six months to a year. Plus, I was never a competitive athlete. But that all changed one August.

I had decided, after watching the Tour de France with avid obsession, that MAYBE biking wasn't so bad. My husband had been asking me to bike with him for years but I had always found it boring and not worth the effort. After buying my bike, I found that I REALLY enjoyed the physicality and was commenting with great enthusiasm about this new effort to one of our good friends. This couple is what I call "ultra exercisers"—everything centers on exercise and they are big bike people. So one day, after listening to my newest biking story, my friend Ginie says, "Why don't you do the Danskin with me next year?" Having been a dancer in my earlier years, I couldn't figure out why she wanted me to go to a dance class. She explained what the Danskin was—a sprint distance triathlon. I looked at her in disbelief and said to myself, *Why would she think I would do that?* However, something about the challenge caught my imagination, and it took me three days to decide that I could do this! I believe that events and opportunities come along at times in our life for a reason. I needed a challenging goal at that point in my life and Ginie was my messenger.

And so I began my training in September. I hadn't run since I was 21, but biking was OK. I decided to leave my swim training introduction until January so I could start out with only two sports. I found running to be HARD for me but I diligently kept plugging along (both literally and figuratively). Biking was easy, down the Burke Gilman Trail or on my newly purchased trainer in the garage.

In January, I went to a newly formed, coached swimming program through a local athletic store. I found out something new: I really didn't know how to swim. Somewhere along the way, I learned how to tread water or dog-paddle around, but I must have missed the day we learned how to breathe properly! So, after two abortive one-hour attempts to swim across the pool in the shallow end (which is just not that far), I realized that I needed more help and signed up for adult swim lessons. Did I mention that I've had a life-long fear of water and being in water over my head? I was always the kid who would float out from the beach on an air-mattress only as far as I could touch bottom. So learning to swim while not liking water in my face became a huge obstacle to overcome. I really had to work to not let this diminish my enthusiasm and, slowly, I made progress. Even today, over a year later, I'm still not extremely comfortable but know my limits and work within them.

Ginie and I signed up for two triathlons that following summer: "my first" triathlon plus the Danskin, my "A" race. Two weeks before the "my first" tri, I tore the Achilles tendon on the back of my heel and couldn't run anymore prior to the tri—so I almost did not go. On the day of "my first" tri in July, I didn't know that a 45-year-old woman could feel sheer terror but, yes, it is possible. The swim, of course, was the leg that struck the most fear. You sit and look at the distance (only 1/4 mile) and can't quite believe you are really going to embark on this and struggle to remember why the "h***" you are here to begin with. BUT I did it. Not a pretty swim; lots of dog-paddlers ended up bunched together and trapped me—but I MADE it. My husband was standing next to the swim exit area and I remember looking up and yelling, *I DID IT!!!* The bike leg was the most fun. I had this greatest swelling of pride because I was actually doing this thing that I had thought about and worked so hard toward for almost a year. The run, which was never my best leg, was hard but you can run/walk so you make it through.

The August Danskin tri really was an incredible experience. The sheer number of women was wonderful and the great enthusiasm of the volunteers and participants was inspiring. The swim, of course, was the BIG DEAL again—this time a 1/2-mile which looks to be a really long way from the beach. I did it, though—again, not pretty, but I wasn't afraid of being in water over my head. I'm very proud of that. The bike and run legs went well and I even sped up at the end of the run to finish with strength. My final time was 1:53:52—a respectable time.

What was it all about? I found I had the ability within to make a plan and stick to it. I never let myself skip a workout unless there was a true scheduling conflict. My mantra became "it's only 45 minutes out of my life. I'd waste that time doing (fill in the blank)!" I'd visualize how much better I would feel if I completed this workout. The physical activity became necessary and important and made me feel strong and in charge of my body. I enjoyed the rewards of seeing progress, even small steps, on a daily, weekly and monthly basis. And I have to admit that I enjoyed other people's positive comments about the commitment I made to training and the fact that I did finish two triathlons last year.

Since that August Danskin tri, I have continued to train in much the same way but now it has taken on a different purpose. Last year, it was all about the new challenges and the goal of completing my two triathlons. Even though I plan to do the Danskin and another tri again this year, I am now exercising because I like it, without a strong specific goal of completing my first triathlon. This has been the most rewarding time overall because I have found the ability to do this for the sake of doing it... for my health, my body and my spirit. This was the gift!

Cyndi Sunby, 45 at the time of her first Danskin triathlon, is an operations manager living in Seattle, Washington.

Once you've identified a major goal, the next crucial step is to create an overall plan to achieve it. Without a comprehensive plan, you may feel a tug toward your goal, but be unsure of which step to take first. That approach can result in lingering frustration, lack of progress, and guilt. But with a plan, you'll have action steps in front of you. Success with one step creates confidence and the motivation to move on to the next.

Both of the triathletes in the two stories above readily acknowledge the power of goals and plans in their lives. Laurel wanted to improve her level of fitness so much that she hired a personal trainer to come to her house two days per week to work out with her. But unless the trainer was physically at Laurel's house, Laurel would easily find excuses not to exercise on her own; this was despite her desire to be in better shape. It was only after she set the specific goal of completing a Danskin and had a plan to achieve that goal that she stopped finding excuses. By the time Laurel achieved her goal of completing the Danskin, she had rediscovered her inner athlete and fitness had become an established part of life.

Cyndi's story illustrates a woman who found she had the power to set a goal and make a workable plan. First, because of her goal to train for and complete two triathlons, Cyndi found herself sticking to her workout agenda. This was compared to an earlier tendency to be active for a while and then slip back into inactivity for long periods. She focused on biking and running at first, because Cyndi knew swimming would be her biggest challenge. Then her experience with some initial swimming training at an athletic store showed her that she needed more help. With adult swimming lessons, Cyndi was able to overcome a lifelong fear of being in water over her head. With the proper instruction, she improved her swimming to a point that would work in the triathlons. Then, when faced with a setback, she had enough motivation to prevent a pulled Achilles tendon from keeping her from reaching the goal. Cyndi set a physical goal and was rewarded with a new sense of enjoyment in exercise as well as interest in future participation in the challenge of triathlon.

LESSON: To lead an optimal life, you need a challenge. When you need a challenge, set a goal.

To live at an optimal level, experiencing moments of flow where time passes without thinking, we need activities which are goal-directed and could not be done without appropriate skills. An appropriate goal should stretch just beyond what we think we can accomplish with the skill set we possess.

TAKE AN AMAZING RIDE
by Elizabeth Erwin

I was coming home from work every day feeling bored and worthless. I hadn't had a real purpose in a long time. I decided to get into better shape and try something new. I needed a challenge and what better challenge than a triathlon? After some careful self-assessments, I decided I had not gone crazy and looked on the Web for some type of training group I could join. I knew I couldn't do this by myself. Since I had heard of the Danskin, I started researching that race. I read all about it. Before I knew it, I had submitted my credit card number and signed up with Team Danskin Training. After making sure I wasn't crazy again, I started to prepare for the upcoming training and, boy, was that shopping list fun! I got to buy all kinds of new gear. This was the best training group ever. We hadn't even started and I liked it—the shopping, that is.

Off to training I went. What was it going to be like? Was everyone except me going to be a super athlete? Would the coaches leave me behind because of words I didn't understand or if I was slow? That day was the first and last I ever felt like that. The training was exactly the experience I had been looking for. It made me accountable for practices. I learned what I was doing and realized that everyone else was in the exact same boat as me—a beginner who needed lots of help—which is exactly what I got.

One of the best things about the coaching is the mental training you receive. You are taught to come up with a mantra, a saying that you repeat over and over again when you are really challenged with some part of the course. Let's just say that I repeated my mantra a lot!!! The other quotes that really helped with my mental training were: "You are given one life and one life only, so live it to the fullest" and "You are the master of your own destiny—so if you don't like something about your life, change it." Okay, so maybe that's three quotes I mashed together to give myself one big speech, but it worked.

Crossing the finish line for me was a beginning of trying new things. I realized that you don't have to be superhuman or a super athlete to enjoy fresh experiences. Everybody has to start with their first real swim, first hard bike ride, first race, first anything. Nobody wakes up automatically knowing how to do stuff. After all, we're HUMAN. Even Lance Armstrong had to make that decision one day to take that first bike ride. Being human, there were times I wanted to quit during the race but no matter how much I thought about quitting, I could always talk myself out of that because I had a goal. Besides, by the time I argued back and forth with the devil and the angel sitting on my shoulders, I had already finished the very thing I wanted to quit.

To sum it all up, this experience was a combination of a lot of feelings: scary, exciting, hard, fulfilling, amazing, nerve-wracking, and wonderful. I loved every minute of it! If you're looking for that defining moment to instigate a much needed change; set a new goal, take out your credit card, push the send button as fast as you can, and hold on for an AMAZING ride.

Elizabeth Erwin was 28 when she completed her first Danskin. She lives in San Marcos, Texas.

NEEDED A CHALLENGE, SET A GOAL
by Leah Narro

When we moved to Florida eight years ago, I quit work to stay home with my two sons, ages 2 and 4. My husband, Max, took up cycling. He would go for two- to four-hour rides every Saturday and Sunday. I hadn't made friends yet, and was not used to spending so much time alone with two very busy boys. No matter what time Max came home from a ride—it was too late! The household would be chaotic and I would be unhappy. I hated going from active, intellectual professional to (yikes) "banshee wife."

Deep down, I knew that for me to get back to being active and to be able to have more interesting conversations with my husband, I would have to take up cycling, too, or go back to work! I could ride 6 miles but my legs felt like jelly, and I knew that was my limit. I did this for a few months and decided I was either going to get serious or be the kind of person I had always disliked: whiny and bitter.

So I made myself ride a bike for 30 miles.

Max and I started spending a lot of money on babysitters, not for dinner or for movies; but for bike rides! Max always waited for me and never, ever complained about how much slower I rode. In time, I became a serious cyclist, riding 75 to 100 miles per week and even completing several century rides. Today, I love cycling; I love seeing things you don't notice in the car. I love being outside and I love knowing my body is healthy and strong.

Then, two years ago, I felt the need for another challenge. I wanted something that could only be achieved through hard work. The local YMCA had a flyer that advertised a training group for the Danskin triathlon. I picked up the flyer, and secretly held onto it for a few weeks. Then I bought a pair of running shoes and kept them in the box, with the receipt; in case I changed my mind. I still wasn't sure this was what I meant by a "challenge."

My doubts centered mostly on swimming. I remembered being on the swim team for one day as a child. I swam 50 meters, and then had to lie on the edge of the pool gasping for air! Thirty years later that memory remained clear. But I went to the pre-training meeting, and signed up in spite of my anxiety.

The first training was a 6:00 AM swim. The moon shone over the pool, which was packed with 50 women—some of whom did not even know how to swim. This was the group for me!

The Danskin pre-race Expo and actual race were very emotional. I had tears in my eyes watching the cancer survivors on stage. I got choked up during the transition when my two beautiful, sweet boys yelled, "Go Mom!" That emotion continued when the race was finished and hundreds of people were clapping and encouraging the final racers. Those women were impressive. All shapes, sizes, and levels of fitness, yet they were each strong enough to complete this event. I needed a challenge, I set a goal. Little did I know how much my life would continue to change because of my experience as a Danskin triathlete.

Leah Narro, married to Max for over 20 years, has two sons, Mitchell and Gus. She has an MA in Psychology and worked as a mental health therapist for over 12 years before becoming a stay-at-home mom. After completing her first Danskin as described, Leah recruited her mom, three sisters, and other friends to joining her in "triing" the following year. See their stories in Chapter 8.

If we are not moving forward in our life, we can easily find ourselves beginning to slip backward or get caught up in negative entanglements. In contrast, goals and challenges bring positive growth as we learn and discover new things.

Leah's and Elizabeth's lives shared a common need—that of a positive challenge. Elizabeth was leaving work each day feeling bored and worthless. Her job was not providing a meaningful sense of purpose or an appealing challenge. Leah, in some ways, missed the challenge of the workplace she had left to stay home with her two sons. She hated feeling like a "banshee wife" when her husband went off for his lengthy bike rides on the weekends. Leah knew that in order to feel better about herself and what she had to offer her relationship, something had to change. Setting a goal to complete a triathlon was just what both of women needed to become engaged on a higher level once more with life.

LESSON: Motivation can come from either desire or fear.

Human behaviors tend to be motivated by either desire or fear. Desire is what we want in our lives, fueled by our values, beliefs and passions as well as the conditions that bring us happiness and energy. Desire propels us toward our dreams. So it's important to make sure you choose goals that come from the heart.

In contrast to desire, fear often holds us back. It tells us that we "can't." Fear can deplete our energy and sometimes feels like a dark cloud hovering over our daily existence.

Sometimes fear motivates us to take a positive step related to our desires. Then the desire eventually takes over, and we conquer our fear. For instance, a negative health diagnosis can prompt a woman to finally make time for physical activity, after which the rewards of exercise begin to fulfill her desire for fitness and better health.

Over the long term, motivation from desire is stronger than motivation from fear.

THE GOAL TO LOSE BECAME THE GOAL TO WIN
by Nancy Carter

I've never really participated in competitive or team sports. Does it involve a ball? Not interested. Does it require moving my body or sweating? No thanks! In fact, I could easily have been a consultant on Practical Methodology in Circumventing PE Participation! I think the closest I ever came to athleticism was watching my boys play tee ball, while munching on Ho-Hos, of course!

Just nine short months before the August Danskin triathlon, I lay on an operating table and had my guts rearranged in the form of a gastric bypass: a small pouch for a stomach and a bypass of nearly five feet of intestine.

Two months prior to surgery, I had begun a walking regimen at the adamant demand of my surgeon. At the start, I could not walk one-quarter a mile without being red-faced, struggling to breathe, and feeling ready to drop. Our hill, only a few blocks long, was impossible for me to climb without several recovery stops. I weighed nearly 280 pounds.

Eventually, I began to enjoy the challenge of walking. It became my goal to complete a five-mile walk before surgery. I did six! Perhaps I should have suspected then that something in me was changing...

It was in January that our Weight Loss Surgery Support Group facilitators announced their intention to train for "The Danskin." They extended an invitation to join them to train and participate in the triathlon. *Triathlon*. The word rang in my ears all week.

At the urging of my water aerobics buddy, Ruth, we deviated from our usual weeknight schedule and took a Saturday morning class instead. Anne, the instructor of our shallow-water aerobics class that day, joined us in the hot tub afterwards. We struck up a conversation and it wasn't long before Anne mentioned that she and a few of her friends were putting together a group of women training for (can you guess?) "the Danskin!"

Hmmm. Is God trying to say something to me? Anne's friends turned out to be my weight-loss support group facilitators, April and Kelly! With two invitations to the same group from two completely different venues, was there any doubt what I should do?

February 7, 2005, I attended my first Women of Substance meeting. I met nine of the most courageous and phenomenal women I have ever known. At that meeting, we set the goal of completing the Danskin triathlon in August, embarking on a journey to discover, unearth, and build in ourselves strengths we did not previously think possible.

Just six months later, we found ourselves at the site of the world's largest sprint distance triathlon ever, the Seattle Danskin. There were over 5,000 participants, all women, all eager and anticipant. Genesee Park in Seattle vibrated with energy. Women of Substance members appeared remarkably calm and steady—and excited! We had trained, practiced, prepared, trained some more, overcome, and bonded. We were stronger women, both physically and emotionally, than when we began. We tackled our fears and self-doubt; what's 16 miles in comparison?

As I watched my friends set up their gear, I thought about our accomplishments. It was not the race itself as much as the *getting to* the race that is the achievement. The race is the reward, the cherry, the prize. The real triumph was in facing our weaknesses, our handicaps, confronting our fears, setting a goal, being vulnerable, and leaving our comfort zone for unknown territory.

As I reflected on race day, I asked, "What did I accomplish?" Well, it was my goal to complete the triathlon in under 3 hours. My total time, including transitions, was 01:49:12!

Beyond that, I've accomplished a lot—physically and emotionally—but my biggest accomplishment is *redefining my perception of myself.* I see myself as a physically active person who has the rest of her life to explore new things from a better vantage point than the couch. I can *do.* I don't fear failure as I once did. The greater fear is not trying.

This last year has been pivotal and life-changing. I am just about half the woman I was 12 short months ago. I am approaching my 40th birthday and know that the next 40 years will be marked by activity. *I want to finish **everything** strong, life included!*

What's next? Let's see, the list is growing. Women of Substance is excitedly looking for other challenges. Of them, I hope to run (okay, run half and walk half) a half marathon in November (I'm a glutton, I guess), climb the Columbia Tower in March, bike 40 miles in April, finish an Olympic distance triathlon next summer, run a triathlon with my daughter, and, of course, beat my own times in my next Danskin triathlon. Having these goals will keep me moving.

C'mon. You can do this, too. You can move your body and discover the athlete in you. This is doable and rewarding—in both expected and surprising ways. Women of every shape and size cross that finish line—changed after completing their goal. I saw women topping the scales at 400 pounds, I'd bet. This year, the youngest participant was 14 and the oldest was 83! Some were cancer survivors, and some of those were in the midst of treatment. One was blind and deaf. One member of our group has a handicap in one foot. Another is awaiting double hip replacement. Anyone can do this! I challenge you! Set the goal! I know you can do it!

> *"The miracle is not that I finished;*
> *the miracle is that I began." – John Bingham*

Nancy Carter is mother to daughter Hannah. She is a member of Women of Substance (WOS) in Seattle. She creates logos for corporate image/communications through Nancy Carter Design.

A GOAL TO STAY THE COURSE AND JOURNEY BEYOND
by Kem McCelland

In late 2002 at age 44, I was diagnosed with Type II diabetes. Things were complicated further when the diabetes attacked my kidneys, which had been weakened since early childhood by kidney disease. The doctors prescribed medications and preached at me about changing my lifestyle. My family was incredibly supportive, but for months I struggled with depression.

Finally, a kidney biopsy brought home to me the reality of dialysis in my future if I didn't heed the doctors' advice. A dear friend challenged me to take up swimming. I had been very athletic when I was younger, but had not exercised regularly in years. The first few months were difficult—I couldn't even swim one length without stopping to tread water and breathe. Slowly, I got better, and by the end of the Summer 2003, I was swimming a mile three times a week. When the weather turned colder, I substituted walking in my neighborhood for some of my morning swims. My blood glucose levels began to stabilize.

In December that year, another friend told me about the Danskin Women's Triathlon and suggested I should try it. The doctors told me that if I kept up my new regimen of exercise and proper diet, I could get off the diabetes medication, and I figured the Danskin would provide me with a goal to help me stay the course. I went to Sally's talk in late March, where she both inspired and terrified me—I had not been on a bicycle in 25 years—so I immediately signed up for Team Danskin Training.

That was a year ago this week. During that year, I bought four bicycles and completed the Danskin (within my goal of under two hours), five additional triathlons, two century rides, and six metric century rides. I was also taken off my diabetes medication and my doctors have pronounced me "symptom-free." But most importantly, through Danskin and the Team Danskin Training program, I met a wonderful group of women, some of whom have become not just my workout buddies, but also my friends.

Kem McClelland is an intellectual property attorney from Austin, Texas. She is the mother of one son, stepmother to two, and a new grandmother! With her 50th birthday just around the corner, her goal is "to do the Vineman half-Ironman distance Aqua-Bike event in Napa this summer, then head off to Spain or France for a two-week cycling vacation." Kem reports: "My health remains good (diabetes symptoms still at bay) thanks to continued exercise (mostly cycling) and proper nutrition."

Similar to how motivation has its two faces of desire and fear, it can also be looked at as either *intrinsic* or *extrinsic*. Extrinsic motivation comes from outside of us and includes all the things that other people (loved ones, doctors, etc.) think we should do. We can experience a lot of pressure to make changes in our lives based on extrinsic forces. Intrinsic motivation comes from within you, from being aware of what's truly important and valuable to you. Whereas interest in accomplishing extrinsically motivated goals may wane, the passion associated with intrinsic motivation provides the energy to keep you going.

Both Nancy's and Kem's stories illustrate the transition from being motivated by external forces and fear to internal forces motivated by desire. Fear for their health and doctor admonitions were the starting point. In the end, each developed internal motivation to stay healthy and set goals.

Nancy set a number of goals along the way for herself. Prior to her planned gastric by-pass surgery, at her doctor's insistence, she started walking. At that point, Nancy's motivation was created from a perspective of fear for her health. Bypass surgery was scheduled to overcome weight goals and her initial efforts to walk were driven by her doctor's insistence.

As Nancy began to recognize the benefits of walking and to see progress from her efforts, her motivation switched from fear to coming from a place of desire. When she set the goal of walking five miles prior to surgery—which certainly appeared to be a stretch goal at the time for Nancy—she exceeded her goal and walked six.

After surgery, having learned the value of goals, Nancy set the goal to complete a Danskin triathlon. Over the six months she trained with Women of Substance, she improved physically as well as emotionally. She moved outside her comfort zone, conquered fears, and totally changed her perception of herself.

Nancy sets goals for the future, determined by what is truly important to her. New goals include completing a half marathon and an Olympic distance triathlon as a way to stay strong—both physically and mentally.

Kem's story echoes many of the same themes. Her original fitness efforts were motivated by the fear that she was destined for kidney dialysis unless she quickly made some changes in her lifestyle. She began to make progress. With the encouragement of a friend, Kem set the goal to complete a Danskin. Motivation began to come from within. As a result of her efforts, Kem improved her physical health to such an extent that she was found to be "symptom-free" from diabetes and taken off all medication. Her ultimate reward included the new friends she made in the process of achieving her goal.

LESSON: Gain control by setting a goal during the toughest times.

Creating a goal during times when the circumstances seem dismal can be extremely valuable. Once the goal is defined, it begins to move you forward in a positive direction—beginning in that area of your life. In addition, the goal provides an uplifting focus and a break from the current challenge by life's adversities. During this phase, you're bound to go through a re-examination and realignment of your priorities, and the goal may be part of this new vision of your life.

Dedication to a goal provides clarity of purpose during the rough patches. Instead of concentrating on "why me?" or how dreadful the situation is, activities needed to achieve the goal can create interludes of inner harmony during a time of difficulty.

A DREAM, A GOAL FOR THE MOST CHALLENGING OF TIMES
by Gail Foreman

My story is pretty simple. My baby brother, 14 years my junior, did a sprint tri in April 2001, and I thought, *I can do that.* I have always been a runner, had some training in martial arts, and a new challenge was due. So, at age 51, I revisited the swimmer and biker in me. What great fun! I trained for six weeks, finished my first Danskin in 1:52, and I was hooked. I enjoyed the variety in the training and loved the positive energy of the Danskin experience. I have participated in other triathlons, but they never compared to the Danskin dream: a rainbow of women, with the full spectrum of talents and abilities, all with the same heart. We serve as witnesses to one another, especially those walking with cancer. My emotions on a Danskin day produce both laughter and tears... all good, because they are so real.

When training for the 2005 tri, I followed a written plan, took a triathlon class, and it paid off. I felt stronger than ever, in the best shape of my life. Every year, my goal is to improve my time a bit, and have fun, of course. I accomplished that for the fourth year with a 1:36. Again, standing with thousands of women, at the start of the race, was such a privilege.

About a week later, I started have some stomach cramps and a little problem with diarrhea. I thought I had swallowed something in the lake during the Danskin swim and was given medicine. The next two weeks, taking Immodium nonstop, I continued to be sick with flu-like symptoms that got more and more severe. It got to the point that I couldn't run due to the gut pain. Now this was serious! Bloating was addressed with elastic waist bands, and life went on. Three weeks into this, I had a CT scan which revealed ovarian cancer stage III. *Very bad.*

I called my sisters (who do the Danskin every year with me) and broke the news. My sister Sandy had thyroid cancer and successful surgery, two years before. I told her, "I have good news and I have bad news. The good news is I'll get to swim with you in the Survivor wave next year. The bad news is I have ovarian cancer." The Danskin experience, with family and friends, was one of the first things in my life that I knew I had to hold on to. I knew it would help me to get through and provide a short-term goal and positive focus.

Three weeks after the surgery, I tentatively got back in the water and swam half a lap and had to walk the rest. But boy oh boy, it was so soothing. I walked outside my house several times a day, for five minutes at a time. By six weeks post op, I was doing my crunches, walking one mile, biking two, and swimming several laps. While swimming, I visualized my cancer cells being vaporized by shining, healing energy—always knowing that this would all culminate July 9, 2006.

I went on to finish that Danskin, together with my sister, at 1:55 and all smiles. Thanks to Sally and all the Danskin women, completing the Danskin remains a tradition in my family. I had tears borne of gratefulness and wonder. Here I was, in the morning light, with all this powerful, feminine energy gathered around me. I had come through an unexpected fight with cancer, and was there as a survivor. Cancer can come to anyone, anytime. Thank goodness I had the Danskin dream to help me through.

Gail Foreman is a self-described "daughter, sister, wife, mother, grandmother, Christian, registered nurse." Recently she's added "triathlete and cancer survivor!" and she remarks, "How blessed I am." She returned to the Danskin again in 2007, the year after submitting this story.

It takes a special person to be motivated from desire rather than fear in circumstances such as those faced by Gail, i.e. ovarian cancer. To her credit, she was motivated to be healthy again and to share the positive experience of the Danskin triathlon with her sisters—a choice which came naturally from within her and was proactively made.

For those who are faced with a health challenge, a quicker recovery occurs if they begin in a place of relatively good physical health. This was something in Gail's favor, as she had already been quite physically active way before her diagnosis. Also, given the power of the mind in healing the body, she surely benefited too from the healthy mental attitude that results from working with a goal such as a triathlon.

Goals and Challenges – Signposts on the Path to Our Dreams

So now you know that goals are necessary to turn your dreams into reality. One of the most important things to remember when creating goals is to make them *challenging, but achievable.* If they are too hard or impossible, only frustration will result. Create a goal that you can believe in.

The likelihood of achieving a goal is highest if it also exhibits the following characteristics:

- **It must be as specific as possible and measurable.** Identify exactly what you want to accomplish by what date so you can determine whether or not you have achieved your goal. For example, instead of setting a goal of "doing a triathlon someday," choose "I'd like to do the Chicagoland Danskin triathlon on July 13, 2008, and finish under 2 hours and 10 minutes." Also, to reinforce your efforts, visualize yourself completing your goal, over and over again. This will also provide some specific details of what you'll need to accomplish.

- **It must be a stretch goal.** Our goals need to make use of our existing skills and provide the opportunity to expand them. There must be a good match between the use of our skills and the goals. If the goal is such a long-shot that we may not believe we can achieve it, it will not be motivating. On the other hand, if the goal is trivial and unimportant, we won't derive sufficient satisfaction from achieving the goal.

- **It must be written.** By putting our goals in writing, we set our subconscious minds to work—a powerful force that helps us be successful. "When you write it all down, your subconscious mind will know what to work on," says Jack Canfield, author of *The Success Principles*. "It will know which opportunities to hone in on to help you reach your goals."

Again, your motivation will be stronger if it comes from within and is based on your desires. Motivation from fear or extrinsic sources may be fleeting, and it is a far weaker force than intrinsic motivation that is fueled by desire.

Many personal benefits will come from achieving your goals—such as increased self-satisfaction, self-confidence, peace of mind, and an improved sense of accomplishment. Realizing your goals—flying across whatever finish lines you identify as right for you—can only prove to be an amazing experience in your life. So go out and set a stretch goal. And when that is accomplished, set another... and another... and another... and...

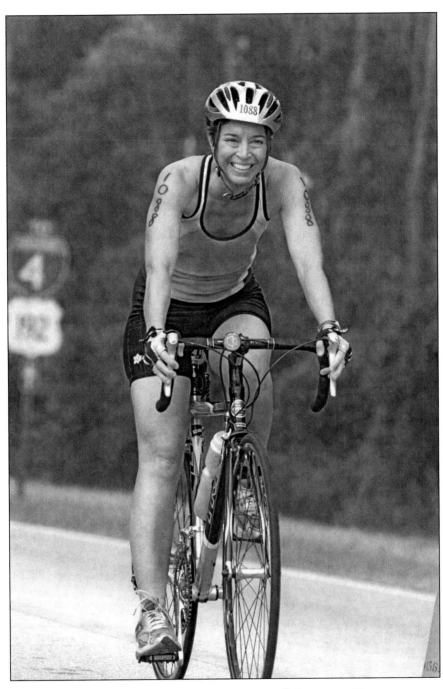

Leah Narro at the 2007 Disneyworld® Danskin Triathlon
(photo courtesy of brightroom.com)

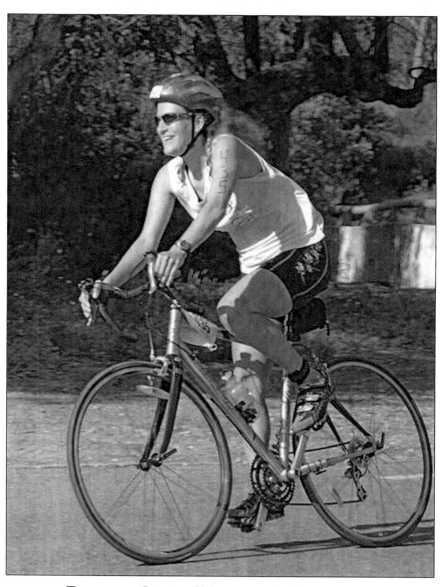

Triathlete Pamela Kropf, riding with a smile

CHAPTER 6

You Can't Win
If You Don't Play the Game

> *"The woman who starts the race
> is not the same woman who finishes the race."*
> – Danskin slogan

Risk is the doorway through which you must travel to grow as a human being, to accomplish your life's work, to make a difference in the world. Taking a risk may be difficult, but you must push yourself beyond your comfort zone. It allows you to capitalize on your strengths and skills, while leveraging your desire and drive.

Can you get through life without taking at least some risk? Probably not, and you shouldn't want to do so. Risk avoidance creates stagnant lives that offer little possibility of growth, excitement, success or fulfillment.

When stepping up to a new challenge and taking a risk, most of us don't make this move without fear. While many kinds of fears may surface when risk-taking, it is the fear of failing that's the biggest hurdle we must learn to overcome.

LESSON: Risk-taking is necessary to keep your life positive and vital.

If we keep on doing the same ol' thing, we'll keep on getting the same ol' results. In order to create a life that is zesty and interesting rather than bland and boring, we need to dare to add inventive ingredients into the mix by trying new things. Imagine how monotonous it would be to eat the same dinner every day—ultimately, this would not be very satisfying. So it is with life when our actions become routine and unvaried.

Some of us, by nature, willingly embrace new challenges and seek new experiences and knowledge. For others, it takes the encouragement of another person—a friend or family member, for example.

We should not shy away from risk that is reasonable. The rewards we stand to reap far outweigh the possible downside.

THE MIRACLE IS THAT WE BEGAN
by Jennifer D. Kammerzell

I completed my first triathlon (a Danskin, of course) on a sunny Sunday in August. It was a day that changed the way I look at myself and other women.

I originally signed up because many of my friends had done it in the past and they convinced me it was doable. My thinking was: *If they can do it, I can do it* and *Wouldn't it be great to say that I finished a triathlon?*

Once I signed up and weeks passed, I thought to myself, *What did I get myself into?!* The only swimming I'd done was on a noodle in the pool, I didn't own a bike, and my running was limited to not missing planes. Finally, with nine weeks left until the BIG day, I signed up for an eight-week training program specifically designed for Danskin first-timers. Our team was made up of four coaches and 11 "just about" first-timers.

We were all different sizes, ages, and physical abilities. In fact, one just learned to swim two months prior to signing up. Over the course of the eight weeks of training, these phenomenal women became my biggest source of support and motivation to me. They were my driving force and became my triathlon family. The bond we formed so quickly was amazing. These women helped me conquer my fear of swimming in open water and push through the burn from running hills. With their help, I stuck to a training plan and built a confidence I didn't think I had.

The feeling after completing each leg of the race was thrilling. While I knew I could finish each segment, the actual act of doing it was 10 times more rewarding than I'd imagined! I wanted to stop and revel in the accomplishment, but I had more to do. The most exhilarating feeling was when I came around the last corner with 0.1 miles left to the finish line. Strangers were lined up on both sides, cheering me on. While the whole event can be somewhat of a blur, the sound of everyone cheering, clapping, and ringing cowbells along the finish line is what I remember most vividly. Participating in the triathlon was an emotional, mental, and physical rush that I don't think I would have experienced if I hadn't signed up to do this. I've learned that with a little confidence, support, and persistence, nothing is unobtainable.

I vow that this is not my last triathlon and I hope to inspire or motivate another woman every year to take on the experience. The only way to share the exhilaration and overwhelming sense of accomplishment is to try one. My fellow triathletes and I agree that the triathlon was summed up best by John Bingham's quote: "The miracle is not that we finished. The miracle is that we began."

Jennifer D. Shiu (now Kammerzell) completed her first triathlon at the age of 30. She completed two more triathlons the following year and plans to be an assistant coach for Team Danskin Training in the upcoming year. Now 32 and married, she is an Associate Engineer for the City of Tacoma, Washington.

THE PAYOFF OF "YES"
by Jean Speigelhalter

It was the Tuesday before Mother's Day (in other words, early May). "Hey Jean, how about doing a triathlon in July with me and a friend?" Peggy, an acquaintance of mine, asked after a school board meeting. *Why not?* I thought. It would be a good opportunity to get to know a few more women in the community, bring up my fitness level, work against a measurable goal, and be a role model for my two adolescent daughters. *Wait, I do not swim! And not only do I need to learn to swim, but I need to master it in eight weeks.* "Not me. Sorry, Peggy. Good idea. Wrong woman," I told her. Peggy responded, "But I am a good swimmer. You can learn. We can train together. We'll have a lot of fun." Although the thought of drowning did not sound like "a lot of fun," I agreed to sign up, and would have to figure out a way to make it happen.

Five triathlons later, I recognize what saying "yes" on that Tuesday meant. I found a training partner and one of my dearest friends. I modeled for my two daughters that setting goals, working hard to achieve them, having fun, building relationships with others, and taking care of yourself can all be part of an everyday life. (Both of my daughters have since completed triathlons.) Despite many sleepless nights worrying that I could leave my two daughters motherless, I learned to swim and always finished that leg.

The impact of triathlons on my life has been significant. I made some great friends, had a lot of fun, got in the best shape ever, was a great role model for my daughters, and achieved some challenging goals. I learned that saying "yes" and taking a risk can really pay off.

Jean Spiegelhalter is married and the mother of two teenage daughters. She completed her first Danskin in 2000 while she was still working as a marketing executive and involved in many volunteer organizations. A stay-at-home mom for five years, she served as assistant coach for Team Danskin Training in the Chicago NW Suburbs in its inaugural year before returning to work last year.

The dictionary defines "risk" as the possibility of suffering harm or loss. When seeking to move forward, we to need face the risk and analyze if the possible cost is worth it. When entering a triathlon, failing or dropping out early (and in either case facing disappointment and some humiliation) are among the risks. Disruption to one's schedule and potentially upsetting family, friends or co-workers is another. In the above two stories, both Jennifer and Jean ultimately felt comfortable with the risks involved in this decision, with the encouragement of the people around them, and they were excited about the likely benefits.

It really didn't take a whole lot of convincing for Jennifer. She readily set the goal of completing a triathlon. With her friends' suggestion, Jennifer was in, ready to embrace a new challenge and experience. Although there were moments of doubt and hesitation along the way, she moved forward, creating new bonds and discovering a confidence within that she previously hadn't explored. She understood that the only way to experience the exhilaration and overwhelming sense of accomplishment was to take a risk and go for it.

Jean's immediate reaction when challenged to tri was to think of all the different reasons not to—including that her very busy schedule didn't give her time to prepare in eight weeks. However, she readily recognized that by saying "yes" to a new experience—taking a risk in the process—she would be in a position to spend time on something consistent with her values. One great payoff was being a great role model for her two teenage daughters, who also eventually became triathletes. In adopting triathlons as a pastime, Jean found that it can really pay off to take a risk.

LESSON: We all have fear.
It's what you do with it that matters.
Use fear to your advantage. Then toss it away.

Fear is a complex emotion that drives us to act in both positive and negative ways. It can have a real or imagined basis. Fear often causes us to react before our conscious minds have had a chance to weigh in on a situation—via the fight-or-flight instinct—which can be good. But when fear keeps you from moving forward in a positive way, it's time to acknowledge the fear—the monkey—and then "shoo" it away.

Common threats to our inner athlete are listed below. Can you think of other ways they may have stopped you in the past?

- **Failing.** As mentioned earlier, fear of failing can be a major hurdle to overcome. If you let it, worrying about failing can paralyze you from moving forward and growing. If who you are is too closely tied to the challenge at hand, failing at the task may put your entire confidence and self-esteem at risk.

- **Rejection.** Some of the most debilitating, limiting fears can be the ones that tap into our social fears: what other people will think about us, what they might say about us, how we'll look to them. The possibility of rejection can even trigger the fight-or-flight response. Either we'll do everything possible to be well-liked or we'll avoid situations where the possibility of rejection exists.

- **Change.** Many people fear change because of the stress that it brings—even with welcome changes such as getting married, accepting a new job, having a child or getting fit, for example. Change takes you from familiar ground to new territory and, for a while, it can reduce the control you have over your life.

- **Fat.** Living in a world where the perception is often that "thin is in," fear of becoming or remaining fat is a preoccupation for many women. Constantly bombarded with media images and messages featuring ultra-thin, air-brushed women, we develop unrealistic expectations for what our bodies should look like. Rather than focus on getting fit, we focus on getting thin, the result of which is often temporary.

IT'S NOT EASY, BUT IT'S WORTH IT
by Sharon E. Best

Attempting the impossible, or at least, the unreasonable, I did two tough things this summer. I climbed Mt. Rainier all the way to the very top, an elevation of 14,500 feet, in July, and finished the Danskin triathlon in August. Which would you think is harder, climbing Mt. Rainier with a total elevation gain (and loss) of over 9,000 feet, or doing the Danskin triathlon?

The answer probably depends on the person deciding to do it. It's true that summiting Mt. Rainier was tough. It took a great deal of training in addition to the physical challenges of the actual climb. There was the ecstasy of achievement and the intensity of exhaustion that came with summiting the mountain around 7:00 AM and being back at the base camp at 4:00 PM. All that was truly great and worthy of the pride that comes with achieving a difficult goal. But, for me, the Danskin was harder.

It wasn't the two hours it took to complete the race; that turned out to be relatively easy. What made it hard was that in January before the race, I couldn't swim farther than one breath would take me. That's not very far. So I had to learn to swim after 58 years of fear of water. THAT'S NOT EASY!

I didn't have fear based on any close call in the water. I don't remember ever almost drowning. I simply sank every time I got in the water. That makes swimming difficult! I couldn't float and never got the hang of breathing *out* under water so that I could breathe *in* when my head came up for air. So one breath was all I had. You might think that learning to swim as an adult is easy if you just put your mind to it. I'm here to tell you: IT'S NOT EASY!

I started in January as my New Year's Resolution. I went to Mary Meyer Life Fitness beginner swimming classes every Sunday for almost seven months! After the first three months, when I felt I just wasn't getting it, I started taking private lessons every Thursday. And I still wasn't getting it! IT WASN'T EASY!

I was very frustrated and many times considered quitting. However, at some indiscernible point, I started exhaling under water. "Suddenly" after many months, I "got" the breathing. I then found out, however, that my breathing was not the only thing preventing me from swimming. There was this issue with my sinking legs. It's very hard to swim with your legs hanging at a 45 degree angle and acting very efficiently as an anchor. I haven't mastered this little dilemma yet, but I found that swimming with a wet suit or training fins does resolve the problem. It's cheating… a little bit… but many triathlons allow wet suits. After I tried one in the swimming pool and discovered I really could swim in it, I thought I was home free. BUT IT WASN'T SO EASY!

My swim coach, Ed Artis, assured me that swimming in open water was not the same as swimming in a pool. There are a few more skills to master. I actually thought that since I could now breathe, it wouldn't matter what kind of water I was in. Ed took me out to swim in the lake and I swam in shallow water where I could stand up any time. The choppy waves and milfoil were a little disconcerting; however, when he sent me out to the far buoy, well over my head, I freaked out! I had to flip over on my back and get my uncontrollable panic under control with Ed by my side supporting my back. I did manage to make it to shore while Ed was complimenting me on the achievement.

The real accomplishment was that I went back again. That time I did better. Soon I was doing my twice-weekly swims in Lake Washington. I was getting some confidence. So I went to Mary Meyer's Open Water Swim Clinics. There I got to practice with about 100 other swimmers of various abilities competing for the exact same place in the water by hitting and kicking (unintentionally) whoever was in their way. Again, I freaked out and semi-panicked the first two practices. Not until the third practice, with humongous choppy waves, did I start feeling confident about swimming in open water with 100 other people.

I was finally ready to take on Danskin! I actually made it through the entire half mile in just over 21 minutes without resorting to a Swim Angel, noodle or my back stroke! I felt like I had climbed Mt. Everest when I got out of the water and I basically floated through the bike and the run. I wasn't there to really compete, but to participate. It was a wonderful day! Over 400 cancer survivors were there, inspiring each other and all the rest of us. There were much older women and women who had never done anything athletic before who decided to try because of the great support at the Danskin triathlons. The back of the completion medal was stamped with the statement that "The woman who starts the race is not the same woman who finishes it." As hokey as that may sound, I think it was true for me and for many of us. I conquered an irrational fear about swimming that lurked in the background my whole life and reaped the tremendous psychological benefits that came with that.

So, which was harder, summiting Mt. Rainier or doing the Danskin? For me, I had to show far more perseverance to learn to swim for the Danskin. Both, however, have underscored my lifelong belief that you can do anything you choose to do if you take it one step at a time. You can learn to play the piano or violin, draw, paint, start a business, change careers, repair a fractured relationship, deal with life-threatening illness, write poetry or a book, learn karate, yoga, or judo, lose 100 pounds, stop smoking, become a lawyer, do a triathlon, meditate, anything! The first step is to choose to try. Next, you need to plan how to do it and get whatever expert help you need (personal trainer, mountain guide, swim coach) to gain needed skills and overcome your fears. Then you need to execute your plan but be prepared to modify it, if necessary. In the end, you can stand on top of your personal mountain, grinning from ear to ear.

Sharon E. Best has built a successful law practice in Seattle over the past 18 years. A graduate of the University of Missouri-Columbia and the University of Florida Law School, she is a retired Lieutenant Colonel of the US Army where she served for 20 years.

DON'T LET THOSE MONKEYS STOP YOU!
by Pamela Kropf

The morning of the tri, I woke up at 5 AM with bubbles of excitement flowing through me. They weren't nervous bubbles but bubbles of anticipation for finally being able to put to use the training and knowledge I had gained over the past four months.

I reached the transition site and stretched out my gear, and as I mentally planned and prepared how I was going to transition between each sport, I knew I was ready. And then, I turned around and looked out at the lake and saw just how far apart those buoy markers actually were! *Is that right? Is that a half-mile? No way, I won't make it* thoughts began flowing through my head. I could not stop the negative thoughts (or the "Monkeys on my back" as they are called by some wonderful tri-women I met the previous day) and I wondered, "What on Earth have I gotten myself into?"

But then something happened. A woman with the number 60 (her age) written on her calf came by and then another with 65 and yet another with a number in that range and I thought, *Look at these women! Look how in shape they are and how much fun they're having! You are only 28. You can do this. You trained for this. They trained for this. If they can do it with a smile, so can you.*

So before I knew what was happening, the gun was going off and I was in the water. I admit, I panicked a little and those "monkeys" started pulling me down. But I threw them off and just kept swimming. I floated on my back for a bit to calm myself down just as I was taught but kept going. When I finally passed the first buoy, the relief that went through my body was indescribable. But then that was nothing compared to when I passed the third and final buoy and I started my way back to shore. I had done it. I survived!

I couldn't wait to slip out of that wet suit, though, and get onto a more familiar, comfortable machine, my bike. All week long, it wasn't the thought of the swim that would wake me up in the middle of the night in a cold sweat; it was the terror of getting a flat tire! *But you were trained to change it... You know what to do if it happens... That is why you trained with a group,* I kept telling myself. Those darn monkeys again. But when I rounded that final corner and made my way back to my gear in the transition area, I realized again, *I did it! I survived! And you know what, that was fun!*

Now I was entering my favorite sport, the run. Except I realized that I had been gripping the handle bars of my bike so tightly that I just could not function well enough to put on my running sneakers! No one told me that would happen. Finally, my feet were in and I was off. I knew it was going to be a tough uphill climb for the first 10 minutes or so. But the cheers of support and the words of encouragement being said all around me by total strangers gave me such a boost that the hill seemed tiny. The rest of the running course consisted mainly of other women running and walking and all of them said, "You go, girl" or "Way to go," as I passed. I realized then that all the monkeys were gone and that I had done it. It didn't matter if I reached the finish line, but I knew that I would and I knew that I would hear people cheering.

When I finished, smiling, I remembered why I had signed up to do a triathlon in the first place: to challenge myself, keep my body in shape, and for my mom. When I was just a kid, my mother passed away at the young age of 47 of a heart attack. I wanted to do this in her honor because her heart wasn't strong enough. Throughout my tri experience, I encountered many mother-daughter teams supporting and racing together and it only made me excel. It reminded me that I am doing this not only in my mom's memory but for my own heart and body. Life is too short to worry about the "monkeys." Challenge yourself. Strive for it. No matter what it is, as long as it brings you health and happiness, you will feel better about yourself. And remember, always do it with a smile.

Pamela Kropf lives in Sacramento, California with her husband. After completing her first Danskin as described, she returned the following year as a Team Danskin Training Coach, inspiring other women to take a risk while tossing the monkeys away.

LEAVING MY FEARS BEHIND
by Shauna Gallegos

I am not a woman who has beaten cancer. I am not a woman who has overcome addiction. I am not someone who has been inactive most of her life and focused to do something many would consider beyond my reach. Those women are in a class all their own. I am, however, possibly representative of many women who undertake a Danskin. Affected mostly by mediocrity and indifference, and focused more on the happiness of my family and other people—often to the detriment of myself—I was stuck in the middle: someone who was minimally active, hanging on to some semblance of health, but not doing much for myself or my well-being.

I decided to compete in the LA Danskin Triathlon to improve myself—to do something for me. Like many women, my days are crammed full of commitments and responsibilities. I have a full-time job, a husband, two children, two stepchildren, and don't forget the two dogs. I have soccer practices, basketball games, school dances. I love my family, and I spend my time making sure they are taken care of and happy (or at least as happy as four teenagers can be). Except for the occasional trips to the gym, everything I do revolves around my job or family. I know I'm not alone. Most women have their plates at least as full as mine—a lot of women have so much more. How do they do it? When the work is done, I can easily revert to being an inherently lazy person. I want to flop on the couch and read a book, or maybe watch TV.

I am also very insecure. I am afraid of change. I am afraid of failure. I am afraid to try something that I might not be able to do well. I am afraid of being judged. I am afraid of looking silly. I try to hide my insecurities through sarcasm and jokes. At the Danskin Expo, I asked Sally to sign a book I had purchased. She asked me how I wanted to finish the race. I was too embarrassed to say that I just wanted to finish. I had to make a joke out of I—I think I actually said I wanted to finish without crashing my bike! It seemed so childish to admit that I was so afraid. But these fears are why I chose Danskin and Heart Zones. The race seemed like it was designed for me. A women-only event, a chance to learn, meet others, share and overcome fears, and reach my goals. And as silly as it sounds, knowing that there was no way I could finish last was the icing on the cake. I was hooked. I signed up the same day I first looked at the Danskin website.

I did decide I'd need help. I can be a lazy person. I needed accountability to focus on the training I would need to complete the race. The training group through Heart Zones was amazing. I will always be indebted to my coach Pam Kropf, all the Workout Leaders (Carrie, Steph, Elena), and the remarkable women on our team—Christina, Darcie, Tina, and Tish—each one of them also training to do their first triathlon. We worked through our fears, learned new skills, gained confidence, all the while supporting everyone on the team. Pam and her team were there every step of the way to make sure we felt comfortable, to offer advice, to buoy our self-confidence. I know that I have made new friends that will last even though the race is over.

Everyone I met at the LA Danskin was amazing: the organizers and volunteers; the sheriffs who controlled traffic; "competitors" who passed me on the run or bike and encouraged me to stay strong; Sally standing in the water with each wave, cheering us on, calming our nerves, giving hugs and high-fives. It was incredible. It is an experience I will never forget and will always treasure. I feel that I am a better person for having been a part of this event. I look forward to next year's Danskin. I will share my experience with anyone who will listen.

It is so true: The woman who finishes the race is not the same woman who starts it. I just signed up for my second triathlon, which is not a Danskin race. I'll admit that I'm nervous. I don't have the comfort of knowing that Sally will be there to finish behind me. But I have learned that "SHE WHO HAS THE MOST FUN WINS." I will do my best, and regardless of my time, I plan on having a blast. My monkeys are gone, I won't be afraid. If I can do it, anyone can.

Shauna Gallegos lives in Sacramento, California.

Clearly it's OK to have fears. Most of us do. But you can't let your fears keep you from moving forward. You can't allow your fears to paralyze you, to keep you from reaching your goals, from becoming who you want to be.

Sharon provides a wonderful example of someone who readily looks for opportunities for personal growth and fulfillment by taking on new challenges—even when risk and some associated fear are involved. For Sharon, the swim portion of the triathlon presented a special challenge—having spent nearly all her life with a fear of the water. Still, Sharon faced her fear head on and sought out the necessary resources to achieve her goal. With hard work and perseverance, she realized her dream.

Pam was not faced with a strong fear, like Sharon's fear of water. For Pam, fear of failing—of not completing her first triathlon—was her trial. She was challenged with a constant, nagging self-doubt as the "monkeys on her back" presented continuous reminders that she might fail at what she was trying to accomplish. She learned strategies to overcome her fears, such as floating on her back when she panicked in the water. She used techniques such as visualizing success to keep her fears from paralyzing her and not achieving her goal. She also found courage in looking at others around her. If that 60-some-year-old woman could do the Danskin, so could she. At other times, Pam knew to just ignore the fears and focus on the task at hand. And perhaps most importantly, dedicating her efforts to her mother's memory provided the drive to move forward despite the fear. Using these strategies, Pam was rewarded with the experiences of taking a risk to experience something new.

Like many women, Shauna was full of fears and insecurities with worries about failing being at the top of the list. She also feared change and how others would judge her. Shauna had become stuck in her life, doing all that was necessary, but basically remaining in a rut. She longed to move forward by trying something new. In the Danskin, Shauna found a safe environment to release her fears. She took a risk and was substantially rewarded for her efforts.

LESSON: Self-limiting beliefs are another kind of monkey that emerges from fear. Let them go, too!

Our self-limiting beliefs are crystallized in those statements that begin with "I'm too... (fat, old, slow, etc.)," "I can't...," "I don't have..." or some variation thereof. They are reflections of deep-seated fears, such as those described above—fear of failing, fear of rejection, etc. The list goes on.

Many kinds of self-limiting beliefs can prevent you from reaching your true potential. For some, rather than move on toward a goal, they'll drop the goal altogether because their limiting beliefs are so strong. Overcoming these deeply rooted beliefs takes work. The Danskin and other comparable events have helped many people overcome these kinds of psychological barriers.

TRIING IS SO MUCH BETTER THAN STANDING ON THE SIDELINES
by Karen O'Keeffe

I am 39 years old and this year I became a triathlete!

That may seem like a bold statement but I feel like I've earned it. I don't have a story about overcoming huge physical hurdles in my quest. I'm just your regular gal who became increasingly athletic over time and decided I could do something I would never previously have considered or believed I could do. And I learned a lot about myself and others along the way.

The only hurdles I had were the ones I put in front of myself. I was never particularly athletic. Not that I didn't try. As a kid I played a variety of sports, but never excelled. I started working out as an adult, mostly to lose weight. I have transformed myself from a somewhat inactive person to someone who was increasingly fit. Along the way, I realized that I actually enjoyed working out! I liked the stress relief, looking better, and friends I made along the way.

One of the first lessons I learned in this process is the power of someone believing in you (thanks, Natalie!). Natalie was a new neighbor who was a triathlete. She encouraged me and just seemed to know I could do it. That unwavering belief gave me the courage to join a swim club. There will always be days when you don't want to run or do your planned workout. Having a workout partner like my pal Natalie is key to getting past days when you lack motivation or the self-doubt kicks in.

I think it took me the whole summer to get over the fact that I was going to have to get in a swimsuit that did not have built-in shorts. I also had to overcome the fact that I'd never been a swimmer. I have memories of not progressing in swim lessons when I was a kid. But just like anything else in life,

I was going to have to work for it. So I was starting to learn another lesson—focus on what's important, like my goal, and let go of what is not important, like how I looked and how it seemed that most everyone else seemed to swim so much better than me! In other words, I had to accept where I was with my skills, decide to do something about it, and have the courage to keep learning.

I realized that I needed to learn that I should not limit myself with thoughts of what I THINK I can and can't do. I have often been hesitant in my life. But jumping in and living life and enjoying all the experiences along the way are worth pushing myself a bit!! I love the process of training and found that I could even exceed my expectations, like swimming in open water. I learned that I could handle the disappointments along the way and that there is ALWAYS something more to learn or work on. Again, that lesson of how others can support you in a way that only makes you better!

In crossing the finish line, I not only accomplished the once unbelievable tasks of swimming, biking, and running, but I also learned to let go of some of those more self-limiting beliefs that just made everything more difficult. I learned that trying is much better than standing on the sidelines or not trying at all.

Karen O'Keeffe is the mother of four children ranging in age from 10 to 3. She has been married for 12 years. Karen has her doctorate in clinical psychology and worked as a psychologist until her fourth child was born. She is from Mundelein, Illinois.

DOING WHAT I DIDN'T THINK I COULD
by Susan Gates

What I Told Myself

You are fat. You are old. You have bad knees. You have rheumatoid arthritis. Who do you think you are? You can't.

I did my first triathlon because I didn't think I could.

How I Got Started

I got started in triathlon via an invitation to join Team Dream from my sister-in-law, Stephanie. Team Dream is a triathlon training group for women of color. I did my first triathlon because Stephanie dared me to do one. I didn't think I could but the competitor in me said, "Don't let her know you can't" and then it said, "You're on"!

Training

Swim, bike, run. How hard could this be? Can I be a triathlete if I walk the run? What if I don't have what it takes? Just start, I told myself. I put together a training schedule. Started six months prior to my first race. Two workouts a week in each discipline. All is well. Two months before the race, I start to doubt myself. Are you really ready? Perhaps I should do a "practice" race in each discipline before the actual triathlon. Good idea. Why don't you start with a swim race? You are a good swimmer, this will be easy. After hyperventilating in open water (two weeks before race day), I learned that controlling my breathing, mental focus, and sighting are all tools that I was going to have to master if I were to be successful in my triathlon goal. What got me through that first swim? Quitting was never an option. I was determined to finish any way I had to, breath or no breath. Imagine my surprise on "winning" first place. I was the only one in my age group competing. Don't think I didn't pick up my trophy. Lessons learned: (1) If you finish, you win; (2) When you think you have it, you don't; (3) You have a lot more to learn.

Better, Faster, Stronger, More

Training towards the goal of completing a triathlon was a great motivator. I'd sign up for races first and then ask myself, *What the heck have I just done?* Then I'd have to come up with a training plan that would prepare me for the race. My first year in triathlon, I just put in the miles for the distance. My second year, I began learning how to get more out of my workouts with heart zone training, intervals and intensity. This year I want to continue incorporating the same but plan on adding some endurance work to compete in longer distance races. I was inspired to train because I needed it to reach a goal. By setting and reaching goals, I learned that I could empower myself to be better, faster, stronger, more.

That's a Muscle?

Sounds like I have it all together right? *Wrong.* One major muscle I neglected to train was my mind. It's amazing how many negative thoughts we carry around with us all the time. These have a way of entering your head at the least convenient moment, like during a hard training session or, even worse, on race day. Often I repeat certain affirmations to get through the rough spots. "If it is to be, it's up to me," "Get out of your own way," "Stay strong," "What are you made of?" "Endure," "You can do it." If that doesn't work, you can always pray. I prayed my way through my first 15 swim strokes at Danskin. Hey, I finished it, didn't I?

Finishing

Crossing the finish line was unbelievable. Hundreds of people cheering you on, feeling embraced by an amazing abundance of support and warmth. Finishing meant that I could do what I thought I couldn't, that if I believe I can I will, that I am capable of much more than I ever thought, and that whatever limitations I put on myself, I have the power to remove them.

What I Tell Myself Now

So as I start my third season of triathlon, I realize that my size does not matter, that I am an age grouper, that my knees can be wrapped, that my arthritis doesn't have to be a factor, that I am a triathlete and that I CAN.

Susan Gates, 47, lives in Glenwood, Illinois and is a member of Team Dream, Chicago. In addition to her Danskin experiences, she has participated in several other triathlons.

FACING BIG PURPLE ELEPHANTS AND MONKEYS
by Susan Denini

I'm looking forward to the Danskin Triathlon as a celebration of my new life! I have lived my whole life with weight issues and finally took control at age 38. I wish I could pinpoint exactly what it was that changed inside of me to make this last attempt work. Trust me, everyone has asked! If I knew, I would bottle it and become rich. I think I finally just hit "rock-bottom." At 363 lbs, my 5' 4" frame could simply not carry any more weight. I felt bad all the time, really bad—physically and emotionally. I felt trapped in a body and a life I didn't want and I had true fears that I would die before I turned 40.

I feel it was the grace of God that reached into my heart. I know He has reached many times before but this is the first time I have reached back. I knew I had to change but what was it that gave me the strength? Again, I don't know but I'm not spending any more time trying to figure it out. I'm running with it!

I found a program and committed to it completely, something I can say that I have never done before. I worked with a nutritionist, trainer, personal counselor, group counselor, and all under a doctor's care. I had to totally rearrange my life. I truly put my health first and *everything* else had to work around it. Of course, this was not easy and there was much I had to sacrifice, but it was amazing how the people in my life (family, friends, and coworkers) supported me. For me, the hardest part of the change was asking those around me to accommodate my "new lifestyle." I thought it would be a huge inconvenience for everyone but I was humbled by their enthusiastic response. Not only were they in full support—they were almost falling over themselves to find a way to help me! It was a sobering experience to realize that I was not alone in my fears that my weight would eventually kill me. My health and weight were the "big purple elephants" in the room that no one wanted to draw attention to because they didn't know how to go about it or didn't want to hurt my feelings. And I just kept getting bigger. Occasionally they talked to each other about it and maybe the subject was tiptoed around with me—but it was quickly dropped. They knew, as did I, that nothing would really happen until I was ready to accept it all. Yes, I wish this "acceptance" came to me 25 years ago but that was then and this is now!

I do know that I am the luckiest person when it comes to love and support of family and friends. They have made my journey so special. Even before the weight loss really started to show, I had people telling me that I had a "glow" that I was "shining from the inside out." I loved it! I knew it was because I was finally doing something good for my body and it was already celebrating. My heart was happy, my hair was shinier, my skin looked better, and every joint in my body felt better. How could I *not* shine?

I have never in my life worked as hard at something as I am doing now. I have never worked out this much or this hard—EVER! I'm in the gym five or six days a week and that sounds crazy to me! You have to understand that this behavior is so new and foreign to how I have lived my life up to this point. I was the queen of excuses. I had so many and I used them all. I really believed them, too.

The "old me" excuses: I have bad ankles; I have short little legs; I'm not a runner, never have been, never will be; I'm clumsy and I fall a lot; I can't imagine working out every day, it's just not me; I don't really have time to work out; I don't have the money to afford a gym; I'm not really an athlete; I'm doing as much as I can; I have so much weight to lose it's impossible; I don't know how to begin; I can never stick with anything long enough; I've tried everything out there and nothing really works for me; I come from a family with weight so it's in my genes; I'm not a morning person and I love my sleep; I am so tired at the end of the day that I just want to go home; I have no willpower; I'm too embarrassed; I don't really feel like I can do it; if I lose any weight, I'll just gain it back; I'm destined to be fat and no matter what I do it will always be that way; I've done so much damage to my health already so what's the point?; I'm so useless I deserve to be fat; I'm not worthy.

The real truth was I was afraid and I hadn't *really* tried. I actually thought that there was an active, healthy, vibrant person, maybe even an athlete, inside me just dying to get out— but I think I was afraid of that too.

Now that I've lost 125 lbs (so far), here are the "new me" excuses… um… I got nothin'. I have proved every single old excuse wrong and now every time I try to think of a new one, I have to call my own bluff! They just don't work anymore!

In truth, there is a whole lot of the old me still hanging around and there always will be. And that's okay with me because I kind of like her. I am still not a morning person and I'm still a bit clumsy. Maybe I'm not a "runner" but I am one heck of a jogger and what's more—I like it! I have so much energy and I'm so happy. I want everyone to feel like I do today! It's a whole new life! Don't get me wrong, I still love my sleep and a lazy day on the couch watching movies is still a treat—but I don't feel like I AM the couch anymore and I can get up off it so much easier!

I used to dream about the life I would have on that miraculous day when I had lost all the weight. How I would live, love; all the things I would do and experience. I thought that none of it was possible until I hit that magic number. Well, guess what? I feel awesome right now! I still want to lose 100 more pounds but what am I waiting for? I'm going to swim, bike and run in this Danskin race and I'm going to do it now! I want to learn to kayak, water ski and rock climb. I want to run, jump, skip, flip and crawl—just get up and move all the time. And I don't have to wait. I'm already enjoying the life I've been waiting for so long!

I've worked really hard but in the end, I can't believe how easy it's all been. Though I'm only halfway to my goal weight, I already feel like a totally different person. I can't imagine what it's going to feel like after another 100 pounds but I'm excited to find out.

I'm doing the Danskin to prove to myself that the changes I've made in my life are significant *today*. I have faced my fears and moved on. I AM an active, healthy, vibrant person and I am so blessed.

Susan Denini submitted this story in April 2006 and went on to complete her first Danskin triathlon in August 2006. More of Susan's story is included in Chapter 9.

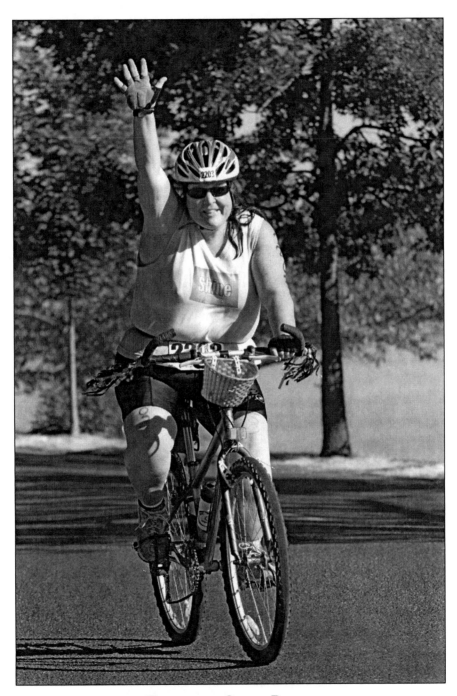

TRIATHLETE SUSAN DENINI
(PHOTO COURTESY OF BRIGHTROOM.COM)

Each of the stories above illustrates the impact that self-limiting beliefs can have on our lives. If you feel that such beliefs are robbing you of your potential, don't you think it's time to take action? If you sense this, negative beliefs are probably influencing your life even more than you know. Because belief work is such an important area, I am going to give you some homework. *Try this limiting-belief-clearing exercise...* Pick an area where you feel these self-defeating beliefs are actively holding you back. Now grab a notepad or journal, and just start listing the beliefs! (For a limited work-life, as an example, a belief might be "I'm not smart enough.") Just jot down the doubts that would automatically come to you in that area, or think about it for a while and then write them down. You'll want to list three beliefs at the least, four or five is good, too, or keep going if more come to you. Next, go back to each belief, and rewrite it with a positive twist. Turn it into a positive affirmation! As an example, "I'm not smart enough" could become "I am wiser than I know." When you've finished transforming the original negative beliefs into affirmations, recopy just the affirmations on a new sheet of paper and return to review this revised list when you need reinforcement. (Also, tear up the old list, and throw it away!) Recall the related affirmation if one of the old limiting thoughts comes to mind. If there is work to be done to fully embrace the affirmation, do it. But know that awareness is a big part to turning these beliefs around.

In the story above, Karen readily acknowledged her previous tendency to limit her activities and experiences because of self-limiting beliefs. *I'm not an athlete,* she thought. *I can't do this because of how I look in a bathing suit... I can't swim as well or as fast as everyone else,* for example. How admirable that Karen was able to acknowledge these self-limiting beliefs and then let them go! In moving forward, she learned that it's better to live life than to watch it go by.

Susan Gates' story was similar to Karen's. In the beginning, what Susan G. focused on was being too old, not an athlete, having bad knees and rheumatoid arthritis. She didn't think that completing a triathlon was possible. However, on a dare, Susan G. began to train for the Danskin and to make progress physically. Ultimately, what Susan G. learned is that she had to convince her mind of her ability to truly accomplish her goal. Once Susan G.'s mind was in the game, she was in a position to win.

Susan Denini provides an amazing example of facing a multitude of fears and self-limiting beliefs to totally transform her life from one of inactivity and obesity to activity and health. Susan D. feared dying, being fat, working too hard, and knew she needed to change her life. Once she faced "the purple elephants in the room," Susan D. was finally able to change her thinking on all sorts of levels and to let go of her self-limiting beliefs. How wonderful that after losing 125 pounds, and still intending to lose at least 100 more, Susan D. completed her first Danskin to celebrate all the progress she'd already made—that she didn't let her size or others' perceptions keep her from living out a dream to be an active, fit person.

Seize the Day! Your Life Is Waiting...

There are so many opportunities in life to realize our potential, to stretch ourselves and become the person we were meant to be. What a waste to just stand frozen in place and not experience all the wonderful things life has to offer because of fear or some self-limiting beliefs.

When we are afraid, the fear can become like a straitjacket on our lives. The key is to acknowledge the fear, know that others are likely experiencing it too, but keep moving forward anyways. Even if you fail to accomplish your goal on your first attempt, you're a better person for having taken a risk. You've learned something new. You've moved out of your comfort zone. You're better prepared for next time. Remember, just because you've failed, doesn't mean you're a failure.

If self-limiting beliefs have you stuck, try the limiting-belief-clearing exercise above. Create a higher awareness of how your thinking is limiting your experience and how you could see things differently. Surround yourself with people who believe in you (more on this in Chapter 8). Talk about it with a friend, or if you need more help, seek out a coach or therapist. Take some time for self-examination.

And get out there! Sign up for your first Danskin. Move on to an Olympic distance race. Climb a mountain or go river-rafting. Ride a hot air balloon. Whatever you choose, look for opportunities to stretch and grow and move forward. Become the person you were meant to be!

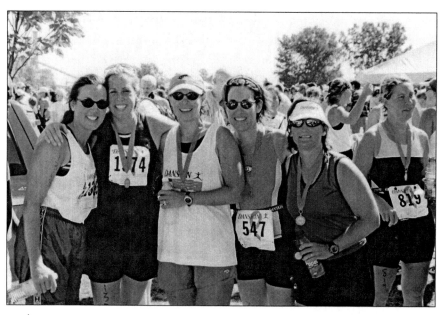

A SENSE OF ACCOMPLISHMENT SHARED AFTER ACHIEVING A GOAL

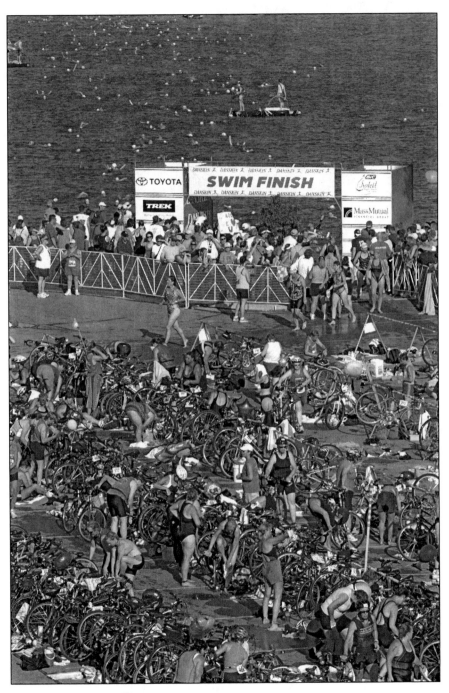

Swim finish to bike transition
(photo courtesy of brightroom.com)

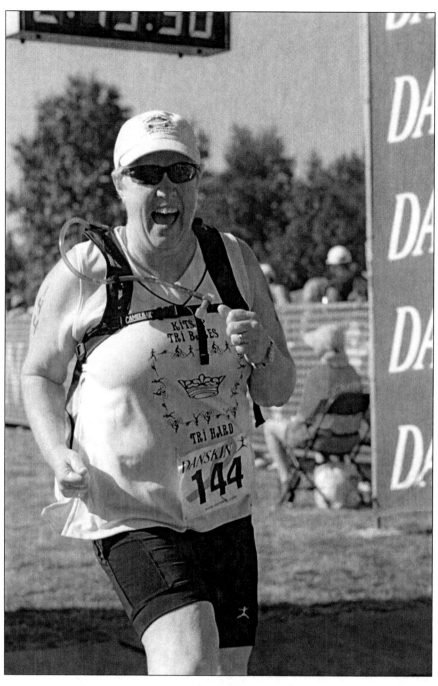

DONNA WAGNER COMPLETES HER FIRST
DANSKIN TRIATHLON IN SEATTLE.
(PHOTO COURTESY OF BRIGHTROOM.COM)

CHAPTER 7

Obstacles – Roadblocks and Rocks along the Path

(You Learn the Most from the Tough Times)

> *"Doing the Danskin was a symbol of reclaiming my body, spirt and mind back from cancer. Not only can you recover, but you can be better, healthier, and stronger and accomplish things you never imaged before the diagnosis."*
> – Donna Wagner

One day, you're going along, content with your life. Then... WHAMM!! The next day, all the rules of the game change. You learn that life has a different plan in store for you. You're faced with an external roadblock that's completely out of your control, such as a potentially life-threatening health issue, divorce after a long-term marriage, or the death of someone close to you.

Or maybe the obstacle you encounter is something smaller—a thunderstorm that prevents your planned training run, a last-minute work deadline at your day job that keeps you from researching a new home-based business, a friend's birthday party celebration while you're on a weight-loss plan, etc.

Whether the obstacle is big or small, how you handle it will say a lot about your character, and can make a huge difference in the impact it has on your life. While some people interpret an obstacle as a sign or excuse for letting go of their goal, others hold on to the goal even tighter—or even adopt new ones. The truth is that every obstacle is an opportunity in disguise, an opportunity to stand up for yourself and what is important to you.

LESSON: Find the silver lining in the clouds that block your flight plan.

At first glance, it might be understandably difficult to view a serious roadblock as an opportunity. Still, it is possible to somehow take what has happened and turn a negative into something positive. For instance, such adversity provides the perfect point to reflect and reevaluate priorities. What's really important to you? What matters? With reflection, you may no longer take things for granted and develop a deeper feeling of gratitude for the good in your life. Or you may discover a new sense of purpose and change how you're spending the majority of your time.

Lance Armstrong provides a strong example of looking for the good resulting from life's most challenging times in his book, *It's Not about the Bike*. "The truth is that cancer was the best thing that ever happened to me. I don't know why I got the illness but it did wonders for me and I wouldn't walk away from it. Why would I want to change, even for a day, the most important and shaping event in my life?"

IT WASN'T SUPPOSED TO HAPPEN TO ME
by Donna Morrissey

I went into the hospital for a routine surgery and woke up to find out that I had cancer. I was 41 years old. Some memories are so vivid. Some are like a distant nightmare. What I remember most is thinking and repeating over and over, "I don't understand, I don't understand."

It wasn't supposed to happen. Not to me. I was young. I ate right. I exercised. My parents didn't develop health problems until their 60s. I deserved at least another 20 healthy years. I wanted my 20 more healthy years. I wanted to finish raising my children. I couldn't leave them yet. No child deserves to lose a parent. How could I tell them? They had lost a Mom-Mom and a Pop-Pop within two years of each other—both to cancer. How could I tell them that I had cancer and yet convince them that I was going to be okay—especially when I couldn't convince myself?

There was only one thing to do: *fight*. Fight the fight of my life for my life. I became determined to show my children, my husband, my family, and my friends that there can be life after cancer. That meant chemo and pelvic radiation. It was a battle like no other. Then the post-treatment biopsy, the waiting game... the word I longed to hear... *negative. No more cancer.*

The end of treatment was a strange point in my life. I was no longer the same person. I wanted to regain control, show my body who was boss. But how? My body—it wasn't the same. It was weak. It was tired. I had no energy. I began to feel guilty for wanting to feel better. So many people lose their lives to cancer. I started to think that I had no right to expect to feel better. Maybe I should just be happy to be alive. I tried going back to the gym. I couldn't find a way to stay motivated. It was just too hard. My body had been spared, but emotionally I was dying inside.

I spent countless hours on the Internet trying to find information on exercise after cancer. This led me to Team Survivor. I thought I had simply found a group of women to exercise with, so when one of my teammates mentioned the word "triathlon," I thought she was crazy. First of all, I thought, "What the heck is a triathlon?" And second, "You want me to do what??? Are you kidding me?" Of course, I didn't say those things, but that's exactly what I was thinking. But upon reflection, I began to consider; what better way to show that cancer who is boss? What better way to show my family that I am still a strong woman, maybe even stronger than before? What better way to prove to MYSELF that I am still very much alive and well? Answer: *There is no better way.*

So I started training with the support of my teammates. It was tough. I lived so far from the nearest training groups that it was very hard to keep myself from being frustrated. But daily online chats helped to keep me going. I'll never forget my first so-called run with my team. I "ran" with a woman who was going through treatment for breast cancer, and I couldn't keep up with her. I had to stop first. What a blow.

Thanks to Team Survivor, not only did I stick it out for the nine months prior to the tri, but I also convinced my oldest daughter and my best friend from high school to do it with me. Just as I swung into high gear, I suffered a Grade III sprain to my right ankle. I was unable to run or swim for close to three months! Fortunately, I was able to stay on the bike. There were times I wanted so much to give up, but I couldn't let my daughter and girlfriend down. Then, days before the tri, I was diagnosed with reactivated Epstein-Barr. It was as if I was getting one sign after another that I should back out. But I simply was not going to let that happen. I had come too far. If I backed out, the cancer would have won.

Then the big day! It's a day I will never, ever forget. I woke up at 4 AM. Knowing full well I was going to be swimming in that bay water, I showered anyway. I ate a healthy breakfast, woke my family, checked out of the hotel, and drove to Sandy Hook, the event site, all by 6 AM. As we pulled up into our parking spot, "Arms of an Angel" by Sarah McLachlan came on the radio. It's a song that helps me connect with my dad who passed of breast cancer in 2000. (Yes, you read right.) I knew from that moment on that everything was going to be okay.

At check-in, I couldn't help but notice that there were women there of every shape and size imaginable. They were of every age. But more striking than that was how kind everyone was. The camaraderie was nothing short of amazing. I'm sure there were women of a competitive nature, but you never would have guessed it by the way they were all treating each other.

The swim took a lot of courage. It was my first time swimming in a crowd of people. In a way, I was a bit intimidated. It came down to the choices of either panicking and being stuck in the water for a long, long time, or swimming like crazy and getting out of there! There were a couple of times I had to resort to the doggie paddle to get my bearings, but so what—I FINISHED! I got out of the water with a huge smile on my face. I was so incredibly excited!

The bike was an absolute blast! I cheered on the women I passed, and some of the women who passed me told me what a good job I was doing. Several of them yelled to me, "Go Team Survivor, Go 85!" At one point, I wished they would stop because I had some difficulty controlling the tears. Not only that, but I was very thirsty since I was smiling so much that my teeth and tongue were dry from the wind!

The run... did I mention I am not a runner? Okay, I admit it. I walked about half of the run. You know what? I wasn't the only one. Again, there were women cheering me on. One woman in particular actually slowed down to keep an eye on me the last 1/2 mile or so. She kept talking me through it, telling me I could do it. She was not going to let me walk across that finish line. She knew I could run. She reminded me to breathe. I know that may sound silly, but believe it or not, it helped tremendously. When the finish line was in sight, she looked back at me, told me I could do it, and she took off. I never saw her again. I never even asked her name. I'll never forget her.

The crowd took over where she left off. The next thing I knew, the announcer was saying my name, "Team Survivor Number 85, Donna Morrissey." The crowd started cheering, calling my name, calling my number. I wanted to walk so badly, but I couldn't let them down. So I gave them the turn-it-up sign with my hands, and next thing I knew the crowd was roaring! My husband ran along the sideline, and I just focused on him to bring me on home. Then, wouldn't you know it—I almost missed the mat. The crowd yelled to me, and just at the last minute, I turned to stomp on it, and within seconds, I felt that long-awaited high-five by Sally! I did it! I finished my first triathlon! Yep, that's right. My FIRST triathlon. I have only just begun!

Take that, Cancer!

Donna Morrissey, married for 25 years and mother of two daughters, completed her first Danskin in Sandy Hook, New Jersey, in 2006. She returned to the Danskin in 2007. She has remained cancer-free and healthy.

SEARCHING FOR INNER PEACE
by Suzanne Dondrea

I was always a "gym-rat." In decent shape, watched what I ate, etc. I loved taking classes at my gym: strength training, cardio, yoga, pilates. One of my instructors mentioned the Danskin triathlon and I thought maybe it would be a goal I could work towards, especially since I was 39, and the Danskin would be held right near my 40th birthday. I never swam or ran in my life! Ever! I did do a little biking. I figured, how hard could it be?

A few weeks later, I was working on the stability ball at my gym, and I thought I felt something in my breast when I would lie on the ball. That night, I examined my breast and discovered a lump. So instead of training for a triathlon, I found myself preparing my body for surgery, chemotherapy and radiation. It was, and continues to be, a road that takes a toll, mentally and physically.

A few months after my last radiation treatment, I participated in my first sprint triathlon. Because of the cancer treatments, I wasn't really able to train the way I wanted to. But even though I wasn't the fastest out there, crossing the finish line represented so much to me. Cancer can feel like a betrayal of your body. Finishing that first triathlon was my way of taking the first step towards peace with my body. The bonus was that I met a group of women who are not only cancer survivors, but some of the strongest women I have ever met. These women make up the Team Survivor chapter of my area.

Right after that first race, we began training together for the next year's Danskin triathlon. And I crossed the finish line again! But the best part was being with all my teammates after the race. We all finished the race and had a great time.

If anyone had ever told me two years ago that I would be a cancer survivor, finish two triathlons and numerous 5ks and a 10k, plus join a running club, I would have laughed out loud. I am now training to "tri" to complete two to three sprint triathlons next season. And to continue to make peace with my body.

Suzanne Dondrea is from Jackson, New Jersey

RECLAIMING BODY, MIND, AND SPIRIT
by Donna Wagner

In November a few years ago, I was diagnosed with Stage I breast cancer. After two lumpectomies, six months of chemo and seven weeks of radiation, I finished treatment the following August. I am now recovered, cancer-free, and I will take Femara for five years. That same August, two of my co-workers and friends, Katherine and Robin, did the Seattle Danskin in my honor. I was vaguely aware of the Danskin Triathlon and was touched and extremely impressed that they were able to accomplish such a momentous endeavor. A year later, they did the triathlon again. This time it got me thinking, *Maybe I could do it, too.* I decided I wanted to tri!

Over the next few months, I told EVERYONE that I was going to do a triathlon the following August. I told everyone so I wouldn't be able to back out of it. I had never had formal swimming lessons so I started classes in the fall. I remember how excited I was when I did one full lap! In the spring, I started riding my new bike—hadn't been on one since I was a kid. I could only ride 1/4 mile before I had spaghetti legs but I kept going. Again, I remember how excited I was the first time I rode 5 miles! I was never a runner but I could walk—that was the easiest part!

Over the months of training, I gave a lot of thought to my reasons for doing the Seattle Danskin Triathlon on August 20, 2006. My first reason was to thank my friends, Katherine and Robin, for doing it for me while I was in treatment. (They both did the Danskin again with me, one as a participant and the other as a Swim Angel.) After a while, I realized I was doing it as a symbol of reclaiming my body, spirit, and mind back from the cancer. Then I finally realized I was doing it for all the women who would come behind me in their fight to overcome breast cancer to show them that, not only can you recover, but you can be better, healthier, and stronger and accomplish things you never imagined you would want to do before diagnosis.

I never thought I would want to or could do a triathlon. Now I know I can! I was excited and scared at the same time but I knew I could do it. Doing the physical part of the triathlon was such a small part of the experience. Being with 4,000 women all doing the same thing—feeling the collective power and positive thinking—was incredible! It's a feeling I've never experienced before. Thank you to Danskin and Sally Edwards for supporting women everywhere as we all strive to make ourselves healthier and for the research that is funded so that women in the future will never have to experience cancer!

Donna Wagner completed her first Danskin triathlon in 2006 at the age of 52. She is from Silverdale, Washington.

Who would not be frightened initially to hear a diagnosis of the dreaded "C" word or of another equally challenging health threat?

The immediate reactions in the cases of Donna M., Suzanne and Donna W. include fear followed by the need to determine appropriate treatment.

For these three women, facing cancer created both physical and mental challenges. How could they trust their bodies again after the betrayal that cancer brought? How could they bring a sense of peace to their minds and bodies?

Each of them found that setting the goal to complete a triathlon—which never had occurred to Donna M. or Donna W. prior to their illnesses—provided a way to strengthen their bodies as well as their mental resources. It was an activity that also allowed them to make peace with their bodies.

LESSON: Reestablishing a physical routine may provide emotional recovery.

In times of an emotional setback, we need something to force us to look forward rather than dwelling on the past. This is why it's a smart time to establish a workout routine, which provides a focus of improving your physical performance and appearance. Plus, exercise has been proven to reduce feelings of depression. Regular exercise provides periods of normalcy and an uplift in energy and mood, so it may be just the key to start you moving forward again. Note that setting a workout goal, such as becoming a triathlete, increases the likelihood that you'll stick to your physical activity plan.

WITHOUT MY HUSBAND, MY BEST FRIEND...
by Rita Neitz Howard

On July 5, 2005, my husband's surgeon came to the waiting room to report to me that my husband and best friend had Stage IV malignant mesothelioma, a rare and deadly form of cancer. After a five-month hospitalization, Ed passed away. The five months were tough as Ed had a new challenge every day that I was convinced we could beat. Both he and I fought for his life and lost. Those five months were not nearly as painful as adjusting to life without Ed, my biggest supporter and president of my personal advisory board.

After being gone for two weeks for Ed's funeral followed by Christmas and New Year's with family, I arrived back to my house that was no longer a home. One of my sisters, Rosey, and four college sorority sisters came to Houston to help me "celebrate" (aka "get through") my birthday weekend. That was when Anita, a KKΓ sorority sister, told us about the Austin Danskin Triathlon. Although I was weak and in a big fog, I knew it would be good for me to have a goal, especially one that would help me get my physical strength back. My sister, Rosey, and I committed to the challenge.

My sorority "big sister," Leah, was a positive influence on me for the triathlon. She even competes at the Olympic-distance level. With a strong background in these events, Leah bought me the perfect tri suit and gave me a ton of tips to get through the athletic challenge.

My office staff got on the band wagon and gave me a basket of helpful items including GU energy bars, Gatorade, etc. Many friends were very supportive which provided a lot of inspiration.

My goals and Rosey's were to complete the event and NOT to be last. Sally helped us with the latter piece and that really took a load off of our minds! We did finish the race and it was a moving experience for us. The wording on the back of our medal is so accurate: The Woman Who Starts the Race Is Not the Same Woman Who Finishes the Race.

As I crossed the finish line in Austin, Leah and Anita's mom (Danskin participant Anne Sigler) whispered that my husband was watching me from above and was proud of me. I believe that and feel his love as I struggle to live my life without him.

Thank you for allowing me to share my story. It was actually healing.

Rita Neitz Howard is the middle child of seven, raised in Monroe, Louisiana. She married Carl "Ed" Howard. She received her BBA from the University of Mississippi, and an MBA from the University of Louisiana-Monroe. She is a Vice President for State Farm Insurance in Houston, Texas. Though she has no children, Rita has one spoiled dog named Jeaux Jeaux, a Cajun Chinese Pug.

Rita's story exemplifies the value of a physical goal in recovering from losing a beloved spouse in a very short period of time. With the invaluable support of her sister and friends, Rita found that setting the goal of doing the Danskin helped build a positive trajectory into her life.

Losing someone close to us, especially when it is sudden and unexpected or tragic, is likely the toughest of life's challenges to cope with. The death of someone close can cause us to question every assumption we have about life. It is one of those times when we are most likely to create the shoulda/woulda/coulda questions. The "if onlys."

There is often the initial flurry of activities. Arrangements to be made. Possessions to be collected and distributed. Friends call to share their sympathies and offer support. And then, things settle down. After an "appropriate" mourning period (who gets to decide what that time period is?), we're supposed to get back to life and be okay. But we may not be okay. We may not be able to move forward. We can easily spiral downward into despair and depression.

Not Rita. Very early after her loss, she used an athletic goal to regain her footing so she could have some positive motion in her life. Her participation in a triathlon also provided a focus for others who wanted to support her during this difficult time. Even though living without Ed remained a struggle for her, preparing for and participating in the triathlon brought Rita inspiration, companionship and healing.

LESSON: When the road turns unexpectedly, find a new route.

As mentioned at the top of the chapter, not all of life's obstacles are major roadblocks like facing a life-threatening illness or the death of a loved one. More often, it's the rocks along a route that complicate achieving our goals: the unexpected flat tires, the sudden physical injury that makes training harder for an event, the child who needs care when your work project's due.

There are a number of different ways to deal with the complications that inevitably occur in life. Often, it's partly a matter of not sweating the small stuff. Expect that obstacles of this sort will appear. Build a bit of cushion and flexibility into your plans so you can make adjustments.

Approach life with a sense of optimism. Brush off the complications. Reframe the glass as being half full instead of half empty.

WHAT I LEARNED FROM A FLAT TIRE
by Deb Katz

One word: Janice. Always bugging me to join her team. Trying to convince me that a triathlon would be right up my alley—the next step for someone as enthusiastic about exercise as me.

I thought about whether or not I could fit the rigorous training schedule into my already jam-packed life (three kids, etc., etc.). Still struggling with my decision, I took a fateful trip to the Canyon Ranch where I inadvertently discovered my new mantra:

The power of possibility!

Within days of returning home, I called Janice and joined the team, just in time to be the 40th and last member.

I started off by going to the training sessions and quickly realized:

1. I really didn't know how to swim—I had no stamina and was deathly afraid of open water.

2. I didn't know a thing about biking, didn't have the right bike (a road bike, ugh!), but…

3. I could run! (Fast, so I was told!)

I trained with the group every Wednesday evening from 6 to 8 PM and Saturdays mornings from 9 to 11. I did this from mid-May until race day, August 6th... about eight weeks. I drove over an hour to the beach at the crack of dawn on Saturday mornings for all kinds of creative swims, bikes and runs.

My ancient road bike, borrowed from a friend, didn't really fit me properly but I tried to make it work. It caused my back to be sore so as a last-ditch effort, two weeks before the race, I did a little research online and discovered one of the "big box retailers" had a road bike for $147. I ran over, checked it out, and bought it. I trained on it for the next two weeks and it *seemed* fine ("seemed," the operative word) but Janice was worried, she later told me.

Needless to say, I felt very prepared. I'm very competitive and Janice warned me to keep it fun and enjoy my first experience. Just moments before the race, I said to some of my teammates standing nearby, "If there was no race and all we had was the time up to this moment, I think that might be enough for me—the training was that good and meant that much to me."

Wow, was I ever wrong!...

First, the swim. I got off to a great start and was not afraid. It went better than I ever could have expected. I even caught the tail end of the wave before me. I popped up out of the water, surprising my family, and feeling as proud as ever. I was off to my very first transition—fabulous—then on to my bike. I was riding, riding, riding, breathing hard. My heart rate hit 165—high for me. I knew I had to be pushing it—kept pushing it hard up a big hill, flew down the other side. I was fearless! Passing by people as I eased my hand off the brake, I couldn't believe the speed I was getting and I was not afraid. Then, all of a sudden! Sphiiiiiiiiiiiiiiiiiiiiiiiiiiiiiiiish...

I heard it loud and clear and it was coming from **my** bike… oh my god, my back tire! It had gone flat! I pulled off the road, onto the grass not believing what I was seeing. I didn't have a clue what to do, I was totally unprepared, I had nothing. I began flailing like a peacock. "Help me, somebody help me," I yelled to bikers streaming by.

Nobody stopped; they just looked at me with sadness and pity as they went by. Then some men on bikes, just out for a ride, stopped… but they couldn't help me because the damn $147 bike didn't have quick release tires… **** (expletive deleted)! So I ran to the nearest house, knocked on the door and asked a very elderly women if I could use her phone to call my husband and tell him not to worry—I wouldn't be coming around any time soon, so don't look for me.

After being helped by one of the race officials, I was finally on my way again but my bike didn't feel quite right. Bumpity bump, bumpity bump. And then it happened again. Another 4 miles down the road, about 8 miles into the 12-mile bike ride, I got another flat, now in my front tire. You've got to be kidding me! I started walking my bike towards the finish. I implored people speeding by to tell someone out there who might be able to help me. It seemed like it was taking forever, but finally someone in a car came to help me again. They changed the tire and were surprised to see that it was me again and wanted to know if I want a ride in so I can start my run. Without even thinking about it, I said, "No, thanks. At this point, I think I'll just finish." After all, wasn't that what I came to do? Finish! So, off I went again, getting in line with bikers from a different wave. No one knew, no one cared; it didn't really matter where I was in the race. It wasn't like I was trying to place or something.

So when I finally pulled in from the bike ride, I saw my family (and even some of my teammates who had finished the run already), cheering for me, relieved to see that I was okay. I saw tears running down my daughter's face. She was afraid for me because it had been such a long time since they had last heard from me. They were all worried, they later told me. They didn't know I had another flat and couldn't imagine what was taking sooo long.

I quickly rode to the transition area where most of the bikes were now back and parked because all the people were either out running or had finished the race. I tried like heck to locate my stuff as quickly as possible, but it was hard because it was very crowded. I finally found my shoes, transitioned quickly, and off I went. I heard my team leader cheering for me as I took off. She didn't know what happened to me yet. I told her about the two flats as I ran by, she was aghast. I was smiling, though, she later pointed out, and she was amazed at me.

I ran, ran, ran, trying to inspire people all along my way as I was running with people who were clearly towards the end of the race now. Maybe running was not their best sport. I tried to encourage them all along my way as I sped by. They were wondering about me, I could tell. I chatted with some. I tried to get others to run a few steps with me instead of walking. Then I tried to get a few to sprint to the finish. Finally, I was back, in record time for me, and I started crying—I couldn't stop. Everyone, all my family was there, my husband, my kids, my friends, and teammates, hugging me, congratulating me. But I was so sad, so disappointed. Nothing anyone said could console me. It just wasn't the race I had hoped for, dreamt of, prepared for, would talk about...

But everyone kept telling me, "We never would have finished! You were great, I would have quit!" And so on. After days, it finally started sinking in. I started to get it. It wasn't really about the race. It was about the type of person I am: the person who tries to prepare themselves for something like this; who was disciplined enough to do this; who got ready and was an inspiration to so many along my journey; who didn't quit when everything went wrong. For me, the minute it stopped being fun was the minute the race changed for me. During the time when I was waiting for my flats to be fixed, I was trying to find the meaning of why this was happening to me. I knew this was my fate, but why?

My answer: Because God wanted me to keep it fun, to have a good time, to inspire others, to smell the roses along the way and not lose sight of why I was doing this. When I get too intense, that's what happens to me. So He literally stopped me in my tracks. From that point forward, I was finally able to stop feeling sorry for myself and wrap my arms around what had happened to me. Then I decided to sign up for the very next race I could. (Not that anyone was surprised.)

Six weeks later, the Hammerfest Tri in Branford, Connecticut. Coed! (I still can't believe I had the nerve.) The race was magnificent! And everything I had dreamed it could be. Talk about fun! And yes, after an appropriate amount of research, I got a new and improved road bike!

Deb Katz is a dedicated wife and mother of three from West Hartford, Connecticut. Through her business, Deb's Family Jewels, she creates heirloom-quality jewelry incorporating treasured family photos.

MY "ACHILLES'" HEALED
by Susan Kane

In deciding to complete my very first triathlon way back when, the biggest challenge in getting ready was the swim. And eight years later, some things haven't changed much—as swimming has become my Achilles' heel.

When preparing for my first triathlon, I hadn't been in a pool on a regular basis in a VERY long time—not since I took an intermediate swimming class in college. Back then, I wanted to meet the prerequisites to get certified as a SCUBA diver which included being able to swim eight lengths of the pool—which I now know is only about a tenth of a mile. Not very far in retrospect. It took me the whole college semester to get ready to swim that distance. I ended up with a "C" in the class. Obviously, I don't take to the water like a fish.

Flash forward 20 years to my community-center pool. I had eight weeks to work my swim up to a half mile. With blissful ignorance, I practiced lengths of freestyle (though not many lengths at a time), switching to side stroke and back stroke when I needed a rest. Somehow, amazingly, I made it through the swim of my first triathlon. Not pretty… but I did it.

The next years, I was determined to improve my swim and work toward doing freestyle the entire distance. As Sally says, it's simply the most efficient stroke to use. (Though I do have this awesome side stroke that will get me through anything.) I attended Total Immersion swim classes. After a couple more years of triathlons, I hired a personal trainer whose strengths included swimming. We worked hard to help improve the efficiency of my stroke. I became a much stronger swimmer in the pool. Then the roadblocks started to kick in.

As time went on and I spent more and more time in the pool, I developed an increasingly strong allergic reaction to the chlorine. I would end up so congested, sniffling and sneezing, that I couldn't sleep the night following a swim, and it made training the next day or two really difficult when I couldn't breathe through my nose. Because of this unexpected complication, I was unable to train year-round for my weakest sport—the swim. I had to wait for it to warm up enough to swim in a private lake (Yea! No chlorine!). Living near Chicago, that meant I had a really short window of time to get ready for the swim.

Probably because I didn't feel I had adequate time to train, I started to panic at the start of the swims. Having 100 swimmers around you, arms and legs flinging about until space clears, can challenge even the best of swimmers. For a swimmer like me, it became a nightmare. But even though I'd gotten into a panic mode, I'd find a platform or boat to grab onto, catch my breath, regroup and continue. By that point, most of the other swimmers in my wave had moved on and there was room to swim—until the best (and even intermediate) swimmers from the wave behind me caught up. After experiences like these, I've learned that if I can make it past the first five minutes of the swim, I will be fine and get through it.

Then, as I prepared for the next round of triathlons three years ago, new complications set in. About four weeks before the Chicagoland Danskin, I scratched my eyes with my contact lenses and couldn't wear the contacts for a couple of weeks. Because I am as blind as a bat, that meant I couldn't do those lake swims until my eyes healed. With two weeks to go, I was back to swimming again. This time I ended up with a sty in my eye! Had never had that happen before—once again, my swim training time was cut. Was God trying to tell me something? I refused to believe it was that I shouldn't show up at the start line. Only after I begged did the ophthalmologist reluctantly agree to let me wear my contacts to do my planned triathlon.

As you can guess, because of these unexpected complications, the swim has been a real source of frustration to me—
especially because I know how much I've improved in the
pool. (I found a half-saline pool so I can do some pool swimming again.) I do all sorts of visualization exercises in advance
of the swim. I have a mantra: "I'm a swimmer. I can do this."
I do plenty of open-water swimming. But all these years later,
I've yet to have what I think of as a really good swim because
of these rocks on the road that cause me to trip on my journey.
It's really frustrating. But it's taught me a few things.

There are always going to be rocks (obstacles) along the
route. Though my swim challenges are nowhere near as severe as my herniated disk (as described in Chapter 3), it is a
complication I needed to deal with. However, I wouldn't pass
up the opportunity to participate in triathlons because of my
challenges. Even though the swim is not comfortable, I push
myself outside of my comfort zone and take a risk. I look for
the bright side. I'm so lucky that the swim is over first. I know
that once I get through the swim—and I WILL even though
I'm slow—then I get to go have fun on my favorite part of
the race, the bike. And then I run and get to fly across the
finish line. By expecting and accepting the obstacles along
the journey, I am able to have the wonderful experiences that
triathlons provide.

The tough part about rocks in the road is when lots of little things
all happen at once or sequentially one after the other. Rocks that, by
themselves, might be manageable, become overwhelming and difficult
to deal with when piled on top of each other. If this happens to you,
get some perspective. Realize that your situation is only temporary.
Tomorrow will be a new day. Go out and get some exercise. Create
some of those endorphins that will help make you feel better, help
you create that sense of optimism. You can and will get over this!

Deb had trained hard for her first Danskin and hoped to have a great experience and a good time. Then she got a flat tire. Next, changing the tire was complicated because of her bike choice. On top of this, she experienced a <u>second</u> flat tire. Yet something inside of Deb wouldn't allow her to give up on the bike segment of the triathlon. She knew she wanted to complete it! And once Deb got through the bike-run transition, she restored her positive attitude on the run. She used her sense of optimism to encourage others. Still, at the finish line, Deb's disappointment over the flat tires and their impact on her performance got the best of her, and she couldn't quit crying. The way the race went just didn't match her dreams.

After the triathlon was over, Deb had the opportunity to mull over her first triathlon experience. Though she initially perceived the result as negative, Deb was able to reframe the experience and learn a valuable life lesson—to have fun and not take life too seriously. (And not to make impulse triathlon purchases, like the bike, in the future either!) You go, Girl!

In a similar way, after repeated challenges to my swimming abilities, I've come to accept that I will not be setting any records in that area during my lifetime. I've learned that it's far better to deal with the obstacles along the way than to throw in the towel and miss great life experiences.

Use Life's Challenges to Become a Better, Stronger Person

As our days roll along, sometimes when we least expect it, life will get complicated. The unanticipated will occur. Whether it's a health challenge to ourselves or a loved one, the loss of someone we deeply care about, or unexpected complications in our daily lives, at some point, adversity and obstacles will impact us.

When the more serious obstacles come up in your life, take a proactive stance to get yourself through them. Befriend yourself, and know that you'll need special care and attention during this time.

Seek comfort in the fact that others have been through similar circumstances and have survived and even thrived. Allow these folks and others to give you their support. Create a strategy to move ahead and then look for the good that can come from the difficulty. A sense of optimism is key to getting through the tough times. With whatever tough challenges your life brings, find a way to refocus your mind on the future. You can be better, stronger and accomplish things you never would have imagined before life's complications. That may involve setting a stretch goal to do something new or volunteering your time for a cause you support.

When obstacles present themselves as unexpected minor inconveniences, try "reframing" your view of the development. When "reframing," we decide to see things positively and look for a benefit that can come from the change in plans. For instance, the thunderstorm that prevents your run could provide an opportunity to try out a new workout video or to lighten your mood and get some rest while watching a funny movie on cable. An unexpected deadline may be viewed as a chance to wrap up a work project that has been dragging on. A birthday party during a diet could provide the circumstances for learning how to attend festivities with a different focus than overindulging on food, or the perfect time to give yourself a "break day" and just enjoy the experience without guilt.

It is through the challenges and obstacles in our lives that we learn the most—*about ourselves*. We see that we can be strong and find something of value in any experience.

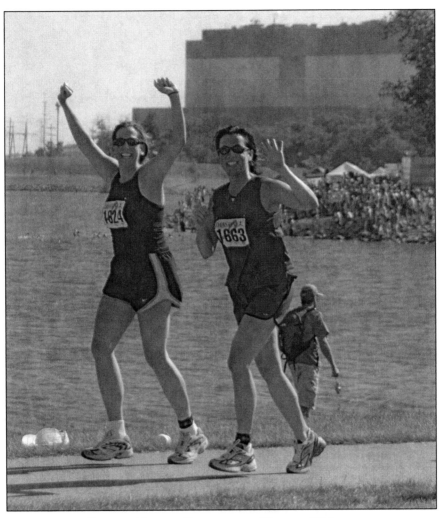

SISTERS EILEEN REISEL AND KATHY O'NEILL

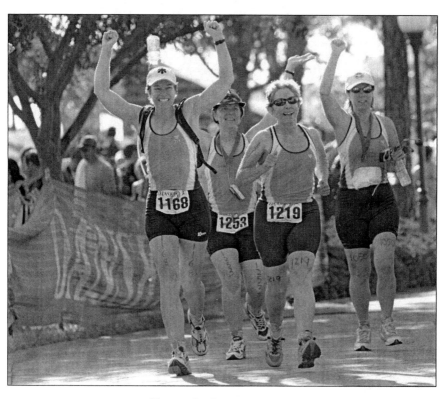

KELLEY'S GIRLS FINISH.
(PHOTO COURTESY OF BRIGHTROOM.COM)

CHAPTER 8

Build Your Support Team

> *"The smiles, hugs, prayers, laughs, words of wisdom, support*
> *and encouragement we shared made my first triathlon*
> *an experience I will never forget."*
> – Gloria Jacques

We all need encouragement and ideas as we reach for our dreams and deal with the challenges and opportunities of everyday life. That's one of the reasons it's so essential to build a support team. You need supporters available who will be willing to pull you up when you're feeling discouraged. You need ideas for getting past challenges and obstacles. You also need people to be available to cheer you on as you make progress toward your goal.

Your support may come primarily from a group of people who share your interests and goal, or it may come mostly from just one person. For instance, when it comes to a triathlon, training teams are a natural source of support. If your goal is to do a triathlon and there isn't a training team in your area, a training buddy can be immensely helpful. And besides, a training partner makes the training infinitely more fun!

LESSON: Friends and family can be tremendous sources of support.

For many who are on the road to their dreams, crucial backing comes from family and friends.

Keep in mind, however, that it's not uncommon for family and friends to NOT be supportive when we move in new directions. They may not believe in our goal or could be threatened by the changes they see in us. If your family and friends support your efforts, great! If not, know that there's a big world out there with many like-minded folks to connect with. You may need to make new friends to gain the support you're seeking.

Still, when they're behind you, family and long-term friends can be amazing sources of support. For instance, it would be pretty hard to beat the family support "Kelley's Girls" give to each other, as illustrated in the following grouping of stories.

STRONGER FOR MOM
by Leah Narro

I enjoyed my first Danskin so much that I talked my 72-year-old mom into doing it the following year.

This was a new challenge—getting Mom ready. We got her a bike, and re-taught her to ride. Then she decided that the two of us racing wasn't enough. She wanted ALL FOUR of her daughters with her. Only Mom could sweet talk these women into racing! But she worked at it as diligently as she did her training and, by March, we were all registered.

We decided that during the Danskin, I would stay with Mom while the others actually "raced."

The swim was great. I was yelling to the Swim Angels: "This is my Mom, she is the oldest person in the race"—good thing she was swimming too hard to smack me! Then at the start of the bike portion, the unbelievable happened: Mom's bike got a flat tire. I frantically considered our options:

A. Switch bikes. (No, mine was too big.)

B. Change her tire. (No, I had no tire-changing kit on me.)

C. Switch tires. (No, mine again were too big.)

D. Sit on the curb and cry!

That I rejected these choices showed me how much stronger I can be for my mom than for myself. On my own, I would have collapsed into Option D.

Knowing how hard Mom had worked and how capable she was, I picked Option E—Find a way to finish this race! And despite **two** flat tires, we did just that.

As moving and emotional as the first Danskin was for me, the second race with my mom was double. Wanting to protect her, wanting to prove she could do it, was so much more important than proving that I could do it. My mom was incredible; she finished that race with grace, determination, and good humor.

Why did I do the Danskin Triathlon on Mother's Day? So that after the race I could hear my athletic, strong, grinning Mom say, "This is the best weekend I've ever had!" Her daughters and grandchildren have quite a legacy to live up to.

See Leah Narro's story describing her first Danskin triathlon in Chapter 5. Leah's mom is Anne Sigler, the writer of the following story.

A MOTHER'S DAY TO REMEMBER
by Anne Sigler

DISQUALIFIED! The word rang in my ears as I struggled to complete the biking segment of my first Danskin Triathlon! Being an always-expecting-disaster-type Mom, I'd prepared myself for a broken leg or fatal heart attack, but not a TKO! I couldn't hold back the tears when the race van pulled up beside me.

Nine months before, when my number-three daughter, Leah, talked me into doing this Triathlon with her, I reminded her that I was 72 years old. Although I'd been exercising and weight-lifting for many years, I'd never participated in any kind of athletic event. I comforted myself with the idea that there was a lot of time to back out before Mother's Day.

The bike scared me more than anything. It had been 35 years since I'd been on a bike, and I discovered that the old saying about never forgetting how to ride a bike is FALSE! But I had to ride when my children gave me a beautiful women's Trek specifically "for the triathlon!" Now there was no backing out! Although I loved "my" bike, butterflies fluttered in my stomach each time I rode. I'd never used gears and had forgotten how to get on and off. My main problem was that I rode with a lot of huffing and puffing from lungs that were not used to working that hard. But I fell off, got on again, and practiced, practiced, practiced. Soon the bike and I were friends and I got younger with each ride!

Meanwhile, Leah, who had talked me into this, began calls to her three sisters to get them to join us in Orlando. They decided to make it a really special day and all "tri" as a family. There was no turning back when we decided to name our group, "Kelley's Girls" to honor their Dad. This had turned into a re-union with all of my daughters and so now I had to be there!

Phone calls flew across the country as we compared training progress and logistics. I knew that for four busy mothers to do this, four willing husbands had to arrange to be on duty and children had to stay healthy. It also meant that Proud Dad Kelley had to make a two-day drive from Texas to Florida with three women and two bikes, and do it all with a smile on his face! A giant wave of support from my whole family pushed me forward.

Then the pressure mounted when Danskin called from New York to tell me that I was the oldest woman in this race. They contacted my hometown newspaper and soon my family's pictures were all over the front page. The reporter talked about what an inspiration I was to "older" women and how proud the town was of my effort. My exercise class gave me a send-off luncheon and generous donations for Breast Cancer Research. Long-lost friends called to wish me luck. Not finishing the race was no longer an option!

We were so fired up with Sally Edwards' talk to the first-timers on race day that my only thought was "Let me get started! I can do this!" When the cancer survivors took to the water and swam out past the Danskin Swim Angels who were shouting encouragement to every swimmer, I was overcome with the joy of celebrating life with all these wonderful women.

The swim went smoothly, and I hopped on my bike, so happy to be on my way. But I soon heard a plump, plump sound. Leah, traveling with me, cried, "You've got a flat, Mom." Immediately a voice from a garage across the street yelled, "Bring it in and we'll try to pump it up." Disney workers began pumping, and hope sprang up, but the tire did not!

What to do? With hearts racing, we ran the bike back to the Trek tent where the experts there had a new tire on in less than five minutes. Back out to the start again where some bikers yelled, "Are you cooling down?" "No," we shouted determinedly, "we're just starting." Embarrassing, but soon shouts of "You Go, Girl," followed us out.

Smiles returned as we pedaled along smoothly and thought we were making pretty good time. We'd turned the last corner, but knew we were coming in last because Sally Edwards came up behind us. She warned us to speed up to make it back to the Disney gate in time to run.

The next sound we heard was an explosive bang behind me. I didn't worry. After all, I had a new tire, so it couldn't be mine—but it was! I jumped off and began running/pushing the bike. When Danskin volunteers yelled, "You can't push it in the road." I got back on and rode it until the tube came out and the back tire wouldn't turn.

At that point, Leah picked up my bike and I pushed hers. We were within sight of the transition area when the Danskin van with Sally in it pulled up and told me to "get in." I clung to the door of the van like a dog headed to the vet. "Please don't put me in the van," I wailed. Then I saw that my bike was already in the van, and I felt Sally pulling me in. Fear of failure and tears of disappointment couldn't be hidden as I sank down in the seat. Suddenly there was a gentle hand on my shoulder. Sally smiled as she assured me, "I represent Danskin, and I'll take care of you—you will not be disqualified."

With that, she freed me from the van, pointed to the Disney gate, and shouted, "Now run, Girl!" We'd been on the run about five minutes when Leah began talking about next year's race. With what breath I had left, I shouted, "LATER, ask me LATER!" As we crossed the finish line, my other daughters joined us. The five Sigler women basked in the support and love from the survivors we honored, the Danskin family, and all the people who'd helped us reach this moment. We hope that they all felt the love that we radiated back to them on that beautiful Mother's Day.

And about next year—we'll be there!

Anne Sigler, 72, has been married to Kelley Sigler, 74, for 52 years. Inspired by her triathlete daughter Leah, at Anne's insistence, all four daughters (including Jennie Curran, Katie Tauxe and Anita Faillace) participated in Anne's first Danskin triathlon in Orlando. Anne was a high school teacher and counselor for 20 years. Her interests include travel, triathlons, auditing college courses, and grandchildren. She is from Huntsville, Texas.

THE INSPIRATION OF CAMARADERIE
by Katie Tauxe

I don't like exercise and competition, so why did I compete in a triathlon?

Swimming is fun with a tank on my back, flippers on my feet, when I'm gliding over colorful coral reefs. Swimming lap after lap without the benefit of my MP3 player is boring. Bicycling is not for me. If I get a flat, I hope I'm in cell phone range to call someone to pick me up. Car traffic and falling off into gravel at 15 mph scares me to death. And "ouch," the pain in my bottom and crotch!

Running is OK only because it's easy to do—no equipment other than shoes and my music. Still, in my first 5K "fun run," I knew I was in trouble when people pushing strollers passed me by. *No problem*, I thought, they would soon get tired and have to walk, then I would pass them up as I maintained my slow and steady rate. Well, I was wrong. They all kept running full speed and I came in dead last in my age group, which the local YMCA called senior women! (I'm 47.) I then remembered that in the small mountain town where I live, there are many exercise fanatics who think nothing of running up the road to the ski hill (2000-foot elevation change) on their lunch break.

I did my first triathlon when my family talked me into it. I figured if my 72-year-old mother was going to do it, I should be there as well. I joined my three sisters and my mom for the Danskin Triathlon in Orlando, Florida.

The reason I will do it again is because of the inspiring message by Sally Edwards and the camaraderie of the women at these events. I was so impressed by the spirit of the event that I came home and told my friends about it. During a Girls' Night Out at a Thai restaurant, I brought out my photos and Danskin Triathlon brochure. I tried to explain what I was feeling—it was NOT the running, swimming and bicycling that was the purpose of the event, but the women encouraging women that made one feel so good. To my surprise, some of my friends understood and they want to take part in the Danskin event next year. We now have a group of 16 women ready to begin training for their first triathlon.

I am 47 years old and I realize that I cannot maintain my weight and enjoy the good things in life, such as a nice glass of red wine and a slice of pie, without a good deal of exercising. Having a goal such as the Danskin Triathlon gives me a reason to keep working out. The workouts are less boring since I'm training for three different sports. Most important of all, encouraging other women to do the same feels great!

Katie Tauxe, age 47, lives in Los Alamos, New Mexico. Married for 20 years, Katie has three children—a 12-year-old and 9-year-old twins. Formerly she was a laboratory technician on board a scientific research vessel and a middle-school science teacher. Her current jobs include stay-at-home mom, substitute teacher and volunteer. Katie enjoys travel, hiking, golf and cross-country skiing.

THERE'S NOTHING LIKE A MOTHER'S LOVE TO MOTIVATE—UNLESS IT'S MOM CROSSING THE FINISH LINE IN FRONT OF YOU!
by Anita Faillace

My husband and I were living in Hawaii when we found a flyer about a small triathlon on the North Shore—NOT the Ironman. We would be turning 40 that summer, so we signed up for the challenge. It was fun to see and experience the triathlon lifestyle. We learned about transitions, including tips like using a water bucket to get the sand off your feet quickly. We completed that triathlon in Hawaii but we have no pictures and no official times and, eventually, mostly forgot about it. That was, until my sister, Leah, started training for the Danskin. I was jealous that she had a support group for training and to talk about it with. When she talked about completing her first triathlon, I remembered how really powerful my experience in Hawaii had been. I knew that I could do the swim, bike and run, just like Leah. Then she got my mom interested, and before I knew it, I was committed to doing a Danskin triathlon with my mom and three sisters!

I really had no choice; my mom told me I had to! Actually, I was glad to do another one. I trained so much more for the Danskin triathlon than the one in Hawaii. I had my sisters and my mom to talk to about training and I was much more motivated to do well. I would call my mom after I did a brick and tell her about it—this really boosted my ego to keep going. Mom always makes me feel like I am doing well in anything I choose and wonders how I get many things done in such limited time. This is just another pat on the back, but it really motivates me.

I completed the Mother's Day Danskin Triathlon in Orlando (2006) with my mom and sisters. I went on to do the

Danskin Austin triathlon with a sorority sister. Then I did the Temple Triathlon with my mom—**and she beat me!**

I learned a lot from crossing the finish lines. In Hawaii, it was nice to have my husband there cheering me, running beside me, pushing me to finish—to finish hard! In Orlando, I ran in with my sister, Katie, and we held our hands up in victory and told ourselves that we are coming back to do another one—even faster! Now the competitive spirit is in us! In Austin—whew, that was hard! I saw a snake on the trail while running, which kind of spooked me—and I think I had the best run time ever! In Temple, I had my husband and son cheering me on and I could see my mom cross the line in front of me, with her hands up.

This has all been so much fun—when is the next one?

Anita Faillace lives in Temple, Texas with her husband John, a member of the US Army. "We have lived in some wonderful places!" says Anita. Daughter Katie, a dancer, is 14. Son AJ, 12, did his 1st solo triathlon in Temple (2006). "I'm really proud of him!" says Anita. Anita taught school for six years before her husband was commissioned into the Army. After that, they moved a lot and had children. Anita has been substitute teaching and doing volunteer work with CASA and her children's schools in addition to triathlon training.

Anita's sorority sister's story is included in Chapter 7 (Rita Neitz Howard). Her sister Jennie's story is in Chapter 3. Stories from her sisters Leah and Katie and her mother are included in this Chapter 8. Another story from her sister Leah can be found in Chapter 5.

For Anne's daughters, a huge incentive for completing the Danskin and other triathlons was that Mom was participating at age 72. How can you get a better role model than that? Plus, Mom's encouraging words provided inspiration to her daughters, as described by Anita. And then when Mom beat Anita at the Temple Triathlon, this daughter, in particular, was more inspired than ever.

The stories above provide another example beyond the lesson of valuable support from family or friends—that is, of combining multiple goals into a single activity to increase productivity. On one level, for each of Anne's daughters, a benefit of agreeing to participate in the Danskin triathlon was that it would increase their level of fitness. But perhaps more important was the *connection* that triathlon training created between the family members—even though the sisters lived great distances apart.

LESSON: "Sisters" arrive in all shapes and forms, sometimes when you least expect it.

Though you may not have sisters by blood to help you with your goal, sisterhood builds quickly among those who move toward a goal together. Whether you're training for your first Danskin Women's Triathlon or working on another goal, you're likely to find the support and sisterhood you need.

CELEBRATION OF SISTERHOOD
by Eileen Reisel

Our Danskin Triathlon journey started in the spring of 2000. My sister Kathy and I were having dinner with our dear friend, Keri Stanley, and she asked us if we wanted to train to do the Danskin with her. With little knowledge of triathlons, but a lot of excitement to have this adventure with our friend, we said, "Yes!"

That first triathlon in 2000 was great. We had a wonderful time bonding while training. Our goal was to cross the finish line and to do it together. What a rush it was to reach that goal. We had no idea that this experience would be as spiritually rewarding as it was physically rewarding. Watching so many women working together, helping each other, encouraging each other from survivors to professional athletes—it was inspirational!

In the winter of 2001, Kathy found out that she had to have brain surgery. Before the surgery was scheduled, she said, "No matter what, I am doing the triathlon in July." Her surgery was in April and thankfully, once again, we crossed that finish line holding hands in July 2001.

We have been blessed to cross that finish line holding hands each year since July 2000. The Danskin has become part of our lives. Each year, we spend the day and night prior to the triathlon together as a celebration of our friendship and sisterhood. We always stay together on the course. Even during the swim, we are never out of each other's sight. For many, this may be a competition. For us, it is a celebration. The way we run this triathlon is very similar with the way we live our lives as sisters. We stay close, watch each other's backs, and know the best way to reach our goals is as a team.

Our hope is to cross that Danskin Triathlon finish line holding hands for many, many years to come.

Eileen Reisel is married and the mother of four (including triplets). Her sister, Kathy O'Neill, also married, has three children and is a nurse.

TEAM DREAM: A SISTERHOOD OF SUPPORT
by Gloria Jacques

The Danskin Triathlon—what an amazing experience!

Being a part of Team Dream in the Danskin Women's Triathlon goes down as one of the best experiences of my life, especially since it was part of my first triathlon. If I were to use single words to describe this race, I would say:

Drive
Determination
Spirit
Dedication
Faith
Strength
Endurance
Support
Sisterhood

On race day, after suffering through a debilitating migraine headache and chest pains the night before, I remember feeling overcome with emotion (partially anxiety-induced) on the shuttle bus on the way to the race. But as soon as I got there and I met up with a friend of mine and the other Dreamers, they helped me get on my wet suit and calmed my fears. The overwhelming emotion that went through me as we stood hand-in-hand praying together before it was our wave's turn was so amazing. I had to keep taking off my goggles to wipe the tears out of my eyes before getting in the water! Over the past two days, we had laughed, prayed, cried and shared together in such a comfortable open-arms way, I will never forget it. I came out of the race with a whole new pride for myself as a woman, as a black woman and for the very special bond that women share. I was amazed and proud to see women from so many diverse walks of life, large to small, young to old, mother-daughter teams, and cancer survivors.

At the Team Dream meeting the day before the race, I really appreciated all the great words of wisdom and advice that the triathlon veterans gave. The three main things that I personally took to heart were:

1. Just have fun and race my own race.
2. Go ahead and wear the wetsuit.
3. Dedicate each leg of the race to someone special in your life, which is what I did.

I dedicated the SWIM to my wonderful husband, Joe. The swim was the part I feared most and was most uncertain about. The swim represented to me the struggles and challenges that we go through as a married couple with young children.

I dedicated the BIKE to my three beautiful children—Maya (5), Jimmy (4) and Vincent (2). To me, the pedaling up and down through the strong headwind represented the daily ups and downs I go through with them.

The RUN was dedicated to my mom and dad, who have been my most staunch supporters every step of the way in my life. They both are exceptional people who have been through many great struggles and challenges in their lives together. They fought against the odds in the beginning—they were chased by angry mobs in the City of Chicago in the late 1960s for being an interracial/intercultural couple. They started out from very little means—my mother, a poor black woman from the country of Panama, and my father, a poor farmer of German descent. But because they valued education so much, they both ended up getting their Master's Degrees in Education. They truly are my heroes for the way they raised our family and stayed strong for each other and us. To this day, they have maintained a very strong interest and involvement in civil rights and those who are underprivileged and disenfranchised. My father, who turns 78 this year, now struggles with cancer cells in his prostate, a bad hip, and failing knees. He walks with two canes—but you can't help notice the strength and determination in his eyes as he takes each slow deliberate step, even though it hurts. I run for my dad since he can't anymore.

Being a part of Team Dream affected me deeply. The smiles, hugs, prayers, laughs, words of wisdom, support and encouragement that we shared through every leg of the race made my first triathlon an experience I will absolutely never forget. Whenever a fellow Dreamer or competitor would pass me on the bike or the run, I heard, "Go Team Dream," "Go Dreamers," "Go, Girl, Keep It Up," "Don't Stop" and "You Can Do It."

This was such an empowering and all-encompassing experience for me as a black woman, especially since I currently live in an area that is somewhat lacking in diversity. I felt proud to represent along with my other sisters that YES we CAN do this, YES we CAN be fit, and YES we CAN live the DREAM!!

Gloria Jacques, a Wisconsin-based Team Dreamer, flew over the finish line of her first triathlon at the Chicagoland Danskin on July 9, 2006. Since that time, she and her husband were blessed with the birth of their fourth child, a baby girl. Five weeks after having the baby, Gloria started running again. She completed a half marathon three months after the baby was born and looks forward to completing her second triathlon.

Women have a special way of connecting that can be nourishing and satisfying on a deep emotional level. Some women are fortunate enough to have this connection with a blood sister, while others find it in one or more friendships. Very lucky women have it in both arenas of the lives.

In Eileen's story, she and Kathy provide another illustration of sisters who train for triathlons and play together. Literally sisters, they have been at each other's sides through thick and thin, including when dealing with Kathy's brain surgery.

In Gloria's story, we see that she found sisterhood in her triathlon experience, too. Though an accomplished marathon runner, Gloria experienced anxiety as the moment of truth, the start of her first triathlon, neared. But with the support of her Team Dream sisters, Gloria overcame her apprehensions and received wisdom, support and encouragement as she created an unforgettable experience.

LESSON: A formal coach or training team may be just what you need.

Formal coaching—for an athletic goal, related to life success in general, or when making a career transition—can play an important part in moving our lives forward. While pushing ourselves out of our comfort zones to try new things, a coach or a training program can help us have a better idea of what to expect and provide ideas and inspiration for accomplishing our goals. These sources of support also provide the oh-so-important accountability factor, which can enable us to stay on track when we otherwise might have derailed.

SUBSTANTIAL WOMEN LIVING
IN A SMALL WORLD
by Kris Iverson

It was January when I was asked if I wanted to join a group that was training for the Danskin Women's Triathlon in Seattle. Some of these women had completed it last year and were going to do it again. I worked with one woman in the group and knew another member casually. These women were not your stereotypic "athletic" women. In fact, many are what we call ourselves, "Women of Substance." Most were or had been overweight and not too athletically-inclined but wanted to move.

My only knowledge of a "triathlon" was the Ironman and I certainly couldn't do those distances. When it was explained that the Danskin was a "sprint" triathlon, it seemed more doable, or at least part of it. I was excited to step up my exercise routine from my usual workouts at the Y. Here was my chance. One problem, though, I didn't know how to swim! "No problem," the group said, "we have women in our group who would do the Danskin as a relay." So I headed off to my first "WOS" to hear about this event. I wasn't committing just yet!

At my first meeting, I was so glad to find a group of women who embraced me as a "newbie" and answered all of my questions, concerns and fears. They had been in my shoes at one time. I decided to give it a try, still thinking of just doing part of the Danskin since I didn't know how to swim and couldn't imagine swimming even one lap in the pool without being exhausted!

Then I heard about another woman involved with WOS who also didn't know how to swim and that she was considering swimming lessons. My mind started to wonder if I too could learn to swim (at this late age) and maybe, just maybe, do the whole thing. I knew I could do the bike and the run/walk. It was the swimming that was so challenging. I thought I'd just take swimming lessons at the Y and see how it went, still not committing wholeheartedly to all the disciplines. As I began to learn how to swim, I actually saw myself being able to do this (maybe not well or fast, but do it nonetheless). And as I came to know more of the women in the group, who were so encouraging and supportive, I knew that with their help I could actually, maybe, complete all three disciplines. When it came time to register, I knew that I could register as an individual but change to a relay team if I needed to before the race. Well, the idea of being on a relay team slowly went by the wayside as I trained more and more.

I was actually excited by the idea of being an "athlete," even if I was a "bigger" one. I knew that once I committed myself there was no turning back. I am proud that I committed to this and saw my way through until the end and, now, beyond.

Coming into this most supportive group of women was what I needed to help me through an emotional divorce. I was able to concentrate and strive toward the Danskin, rather than sitting at home wondering where my life was going now that I was single again, older (I just turned 50) and raising a teenager.

The training that our group had set up was awesome. We took clinics, hired private coaches and, lo and behold, I eventually was able to swim the half mile in training (maybe not technically correct or with speed, but I could do it). We had a practice tri four weeks before the Danskin. My times weren't great but I did manage to complete it. Swimming the half mile took 41 minutes, the biking portion was 1 hour and 10 minutes, and my shortened walk (due to my recently injured knee) took 44 minutes. I was pumped and excited and proud of what I was ready to accomplish.

The day finally came and there I was up very early on a beautiful Sunday morning to complete the amazing event, the culmination of all that training. We had been there the day before to rack our bikes and check out the layout. I was a little nervous but comforted by our WOS group and all the support people who came to cheer us on.

Now here is the most amazing part! I was in the transition area, getting my gear set up. The two women next to me started talking and we exchanged pleasantries. We shared how nervous we were, that this was our first time, our age (we were in the 50-54 age group) and such. We gave each other hugs, and as I stepped back, I realized that the woman in front of me looked like someone I once knew. Not being able to figure out who, I asked her what her name was. When she told me, it was an "oh my God!" moment. Standing in front of me was my college roommate. (We had gone to school together in Minnesota.) I hadn't seen her for over 25 years! It was so strange. We caught up a little, but didn't have much time before our swim wave started. I was amazed that this had happened. It helped me set aside all the nervousness I was feeling for the swim portion.

So in the water I went and promptly got a mouthful because of all the waves in the water. I struggled to remember all I had learned about swimming in open water. The best piece of advice was to relax and take it easy. I wasn't going to be first, I just needed to finish the swim and I knew I would be okay. So swim I did. Head out of the water, head in the water, feeling the glide for a bit until another wave of women came over me. I felt like it was taking me forever and I would never reach the finish line that was so far in front of me. The one thing I did when I started the swim was to set the time on my heart-rate monitor. As I came out of the swim, I glanced down at my time and another "oh my God" moment. I had just swum the half mile in 34 minutes (7 minutes faster than my practice tri). I was so elated. I ran to my bike and ran into my college friend long enough to say hi and good luck. As I was putting on my shoes, I fell back on my leg and felt my knee tweak. Oh great, I thought, just what I needed. I ignored the pain and hopped on my bike.

The bike portion was beautiful as the sky was so blue and the temperature not too hot. It was an easy bike ride although once again, I felt like I was slow. Still I relished in the fact that I was even doing this. The cheers from all the people on the sidelines were so encouraging. No one had ever cheered for me like that before!

Back at the bike transition, I was now poised to start the run. I wanted to be like everyone else and run, but my knee sure hurt. I did the best I could with the pain I had. My whole left side of my body was screaming at me to stop but I didn't. I couldn't. I was too near the end. I just kept going and going. As I got near the finish, I could hear the crowd cheer. So many people were waving me on! As I came down the finish shoot, I so wanted to be running across the finish line; however, as I started to run, my calf started to cramp and I had to back off (damn that "Exercise God," it wasn't stopping me now!). And as I crossed that finish line, a wave of emotion hit me that I actually finished this and was not last and I was proud of myself. It was so emotional for me that I just couldn't hold back the tears under my sunglasses. I did it and I liked it!! My goal was to finish in under 3 hours and I did it in 2 hours, 47 minutes. I couldn't believe it. I felt like a real athlete! Who knew at 50 years old I would become an athlete! Through the invaluable support of WOS, I found my inner athlete.

Kris Iverson, a mother, triathlete and proud member of Women of Substance, *works for an insurance agency.*

WITH THE HELP OF MY TEAM
by Michiele Shaw

I retired almost two years, ago at the age of 54, and moved from Louisiana back to my home in Washington State. About six months after the move, I read an article in our county paper, reporting on a group of local women called the "TriBabes." They were a very diverse group of women who got together annually to train for the Danskin Triathlon. Since most of them had no prior tri experience whatsoever, I could see I was a perfect candidate to join the team. I tracked down their leader, Lisa Ballou, on the Internet and asked to be included.

Sure enough, I heard from Lisa and, voila, I was a "newbie" TriBabe! I went out and bought a bicycle, and signed up at the local "Y" for swimming lessons. Lisa started sending us our training programs each week, and we soon experienced our first BRICK. Actually, I missed the first one, as I was in bed with back spasms. When I made the second one, I came in last out of the 93 women participating, and even managed to fall off my bike into a ditch, while standing still. I remember thinking, "Well, it can't really get much worse, so I might as well stick with it." By the way, I still have bruises on the insides of my thighs from the fall, a constant reminder of the triumph of desire over common sense.

I took six weeks of swimming classes, then worked out at the "Y" two days a week. My first week, I couldn't swim one length of the pool without stopping for several minutes to rest. I wasn't able to run an entire lap at the local school track. I was completely daunted by the slightest hill on my bike. But over time a miracle happened, and I got a little stronger every week. By the time Lisa got us to the event weekend, I was completely confident I would finish.

My goal was to come in under 2-1/2 hours. I came in at 2 hours and 2 minutes. I remember thinking that if I could get through the swim, I would not actually die. When I finished, I knew I was hooked on triathlon. The atmosphere at the Danskin was inspirational—5,000 women "competing" but not competitive, each one with a personal goal. All of our TriBabes finished, a testimony to our great coach Lisa.

I realize that in the big scheme of things, my finishing a sprint triathlon will not create a ripple in the world. Still, I am proud of starting something I wasn't at all sure I could finish, but finishing nonetheless. I'm proud of being a part of the TriBabe team. I'm proud that several of my friends have asked to do it with me next year, because they are emboldened by my success.

Michiele Shaw completed her first Danskin Triathlon in 2006. The following year, she took 14 minutes off her time from the previous year. Between her first and second triathlons, she also completed her first marathon. "Holy cow!" she says.

Perhaps surprisingly, many of the women who do the Danskin triathlon do so without formal training. However, I have personally found triathlon training to be invaluable, and liked it so much, in fact, that I eventually became a trainer myself. There are so many things you learn along the way during athletic training that help you achieve your goal—from how to handle specific segments of your competition (like transitions at a triathlon) to refining your technique in your sport. Are you looking for a training team, coach or program that supports an upcoming athletic event on your calendar? You may easily find it on the event site itself. Do an Internet search. For triathlons, check sources on the Web through USA Triathlon or your area's local triathlon clubs.

Some especially effective programs for the Danskin event include Team Danskin WTS Training (the official training program of the Danskin Triathlon) through Heart Zones USA, Team Dream (a Chicago-area training team for women of color), Women of Substance (WOS) as well as TriBabes in the Seattle area.

Kris's story illustrates the positive benefits that come from building a strong support team for one's first triathlon efforts. As a member of Women of Substance (WOS), she enjoyed the "sisterhood" and bonding that comes from a group of women working together toward common goals. In addition, the somewhat informal team recognized the need for formal training and coaching. They attended skills clinics together and hired professional coaches for the team. As a result, they developed skills and confidence. Because of the example of her team members and the formal coaching she received, Kris accomplished what she never otherwise would have considered—completing all THREE parts of the race rather than being on a relay team.

In addition to the fitness benefits Kris gained from her team and coaching, she also realized an unexpected benefit of her training team sisterhood—support she needed during her divorce. The icing on the cake was recognizing her college roommate at the race after 25 years!

Similarly, a training team (and the formal coaching it offered) was critical to Michiele, for it enabled this woman to finish something that seemed possibly beyond her. In her early days of training, Michiele was the last one to finish in practice and even fell off her bike. Yet, through the training team, she gained the confidence to not only complete her first triathlon, but also to complete a marathon as well.

LESSON: Ask for what you want.

The people around us—who love and support us—are not mind-readers. Therefore, the best thing we can do is to be specific by asking for exactly what we want and need from them. This gives our supporters an opportunity to meet our needs. They can also feel good that they've done something that feels good to us.

When a goal is significant to us, it's an especially important time to seek out, ask for, and accept help and support from others.

MY FIRST KISS
by Susan Martini, M.D.

Now that it's been over a month since I finished my first Danskin, I probably have a better perspective on the whole nine and a half months experience of getting ready for my first triathlon. I certainly feel different now, a month later, than I did the day after the event.

I now have different priorities than during the triathlon in July, but am glad I had the experience. I hope I can do more in the future. But it's kind of like your first kiss or bringing your first child into the world. The first was really exciting and I'll never forget it. Now that I look back, I can't remember the real reason I committed to doing it. I think it was to try something that seemed really hard, and to discipline myself to do something that required improvement, but also help from others.

The thing that made all the difference was the Team Danskin Training group, and how we wanted everyone to do well and to have fun. We were a diverse group of women who really didn't know each other, but respected each other's goals and different reasons for doing it. It was really nice to see everyone improve each week physically and in confidence. Friendships developed just through one common goal. It was such a supportive, positive environment. The other truly unique experience for me was the nurturing experience for each other, which is nice for adult women. Usually, through my job and my role in the home as a wife and mother, I do most of the nurturing. With the training team, it was nice to have other women who truly gave their time without compensation—just for you, to see you do better and achieve a dream.

What did I learn personally? I learned that it's never too late to develop a totally new interest. I learned to focus but also to ask for help and be able to accept that help. I also learned that after months of preparation, there would still be hurdles. There would be unplanned muscle pulls, excessive heat and wind, and even though I thought I knew exactly how I would complete this thing, I really didn't. That's because those external forces would take a toll. I just had to keep looking ahead, staying positive and putting one foot in front of each other while listening to my body. By doing so, I would finish the thing I set out to do. Not in the time I wanted, and not with any fanfare. But I would finish.

The last thing I learned was how supportive my family was with my dream... just because it was mine. They understood when I left early and they had dinner without me. They knew how important my goal was to me so they would not ever complain. I was astounded how proud my oldest daughter was that I was preparing for the triathlon and that I completed it. My 21-year-old daughter told all her friends and their parents about my accomplishment. She was really proud of me. That was really nice.

Now that I had this first kiss, it's time for me to encourage others, tell them how great it was, and to help them along their way. I'm glad this first experience was just with women, for women.

Susan Martini, a pediatrician, celebrated her 25th wedding anniversary while training for her first Danskin triathlon. She is the mother of two college-aged daughters. Susan and her husband, who is also a doctor, recently relocated from Park Ridge, Illinois to Salt Lake City, Utah, to, among other reasons, indulge their passion for mountains.

There is a time to give—and a time to accept help. Learn to ask for help when you need it and to graciously accept it from others.

Susan began training on her own over nine months in advance of the Chicagoland Danskin. Though she built an impressive base of aerobic fitness, Susan realized she needed more from the triathlon training experience.

She sought out a training group to gain more knowledge about training and to gain a better grasp of what to expect at the triathlon. Susan was also looking to share her experience with others. She reached out for help—asked for help—which is something we as women can find difficult. We readily spend so much time taking care of others' needs, but may find it difficult to ask for help and to accept it for ourselves.

In addition to the support of her training, Susan also felt supported by her family. She heard no complaints when she'd go out for training, and wasn't at home at the dinner table with the others during the triathlon preparation period. After the race, her oldest daughter was so proud of her mom, in fact, that she spread the word to her friends and their families about her mom becoming a triathlete.

LESSON: There is an important place for women-only events.

A recurring theme from women who've done Danskin races is the special atmosphere of support and encouragement that exists at these women-only triathlons. Participants walk away feeling proud to be women.

For anyone who has had any doubts about the value of a women-only event, brush them away. The fact is that as a participant in a Danskin race, women swim, bike and run the distance. They don't have to apologize for doing this in an environment that is supportive and encouraging. How wonderful it is for the participants to have a safe environment in which to experiment and find out what they're capable of.

Women-only events are needed and are important.

KALEIDOSCOPE
by Tekla McInerney

We were as different as we were the same. Snapshots of our lives included:

- Standing at the edge of the pond in her daughter's white plastic flip-flops with floral appliqués
- Riding a bike that arrived at practice in a tote bag and required assembly
- Running in the rain and sharing stories of full-support bras and less-than-supportive husbands
- Some with long-time marriages, some with two-year-olds, a lesbian with grandchildren
- Thirty-five years ago, one petitioned her high school for a girls' soccer team
- Buying her first pair of running shoes this past spring

Though we appear to be dissimilar, we are one. We are Danskin triathletes.

Three of us completed our first Danskin that summer. The following winter we decided to invite a few friends to train with us. On a cold Saturday morning in June, a group of seven women gathered at a local track, introduced ourselves, and began an incredible journey that has yet to end.

Two of us created a workout plan and shared it with the group; some women hung it on their fridge and checked off each day, others squeezed in a run or a bike when they found a free minute. But we met as a group on Wednesdays after work and on Saturday mornings for the 10 weeks before the New England Danskin in July.

Nearly every open-water swim involved trespassing beyond Residents Only signs. We ran and biked up roads with "hill" and "mountain" in their names. We practiced transitions in the privacy of driveways and moved up to public beaches and town greens. Email with subject lines like "Kudos to lanes 5 and 6" and "Stormy Wednesday" kept us in touch.

On race day, we each broke personal records, surpassed individual goals, and finished the race running. We shaved 4 minutes off our swim and never walked the bike. Our partners cheered at the finish line. Our mothers came. We're talking about next year's Danskin. We're also talking about running a 10k, a half-marathon, and long-distance biking. "Nearly a dozen" was a recent email subject line. Our group is growing!

Tekla McInerney is from Florence, Massachusetts. She is the Director of Publications for Mount Holyoke College, the oldest of the Seven Sisters colleges. Tekla's update on the team included, "Our team has a name! We are the Femme Brulées. You can't miss us at local races, our team shirts emblazoned with hot pink flames. As promised, team members have gone on to complete 10Ks, a century ride, the New York City Marathon and more. Danskin remains the favorite."

The story above is a composite of many voices. Women's voices. Voices as unique as the participants to whom they belonged. Yet, all the same. By including these diverse yet harmonious voices, Tekla's story captures some of the magic and wonder of a women-only event.

After doing seven Danskin triathlons, I did my first coed Olympic distance triathlon. Being part of the oldest wave of women Olympic-distance triathletes, I was followed by the youngest sprint-distance male athletes. They quickly overtook me, swam on top of me, el-bowed me. Not intentionally, of course. It was just part of their competitive nature. If that had been my first triathlon experience, I probably would not have completed the triathlon, because of feeling overwhelmed and losing my confidence. Although women pass other women at the Danskin, whether that be on the swim, bike course or run, you'll always find it to be a respectful environment.

Yes, the world is made up of both women and men. Yes, we must work together, play together, co-exist, etc. But there is a need for women-only events and women's support structures.

Differences between men and women exist, in the way we think, communicate and prioritize. There is a value in feeling connected to others who share similar characteristics and attributes. At women-only events, there is a sense of togetherness, of support, and of shar-ing. This enables women to discover new facets of themselves and to reclaim parts that have been temporarily lost.

Life Is Much Better When Someone Shares the Flight

There are many benefits to be realized when we have others along for support. Oftentimes, we could go it alone, but what fun would that be? Aside from the enjoyment that being with others brings, camaraderie also provides:

- **Motivation:** We are far more likely to stick to our goals when we are working with a coach, buddy or training program.

- **Accountability:** Those on our "support team" will help ensure that we do what we've planned.

- **Encouragement:** When the going gets tough, isn't it nice to know there's someone there to help you get through it?

- **Support:** During life's toughest challenges (like those described in Chapter 7), having appropriate support may be crucial to maintaining forward motion.

Possible sources for members of your support team are varied. It may include a lifelong friend, family members, or a training program for people with goals similar to your own. Working together to achieve a goal creates strong bonds, builds trust, and draws collective wisdom—the whole is better and stronger than the sum of its parts!

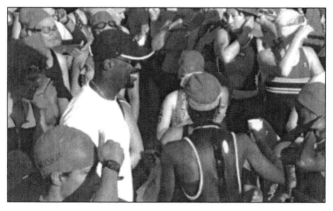

TEAM DREAM DIRECTOR DERRICK MILLIGAN
WITH TEAM DREAM MEMBERS

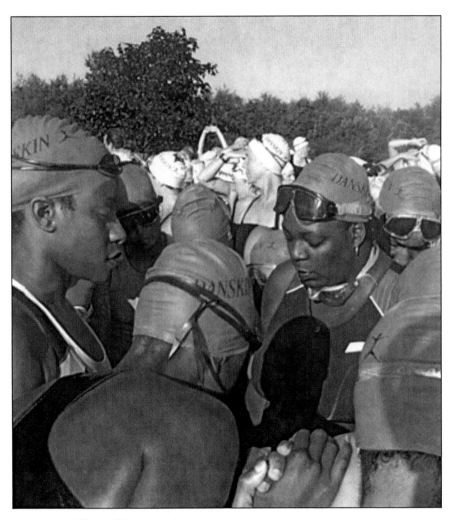

Team Dream members share a quiet moment.

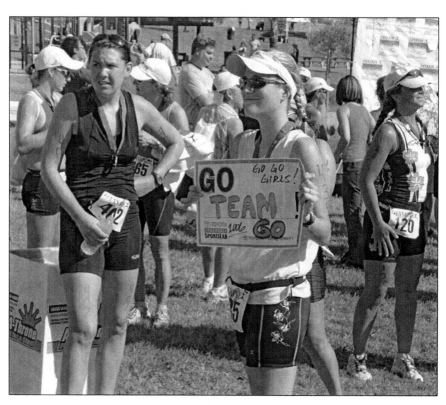

Pam Kropf supports her team at the finish line.

Chapter 9

Giving Back

> *"I had learned things the hard way and I wanted to share my 'what not to do' experiences with other women so they wouldn't have to go through the same lessons unnecessarily."*
> – Susan Farago

As the saying goes, "Love makes the world go around," and it's true. So no matter where you are in the journey to your goal, consider how you might give back. You've certainly learned a lot along your life path, and probably didn't do it alone. How can you help make the world a better place by helping others like someone has helped you? By giving back, you'll reap rewards far beyond any time or energy you invest.

There are plenty of ways to give. You might volunteer your time to an organization devoted to your favorite cause. You could share what you've learned in life with someone else one-on-one. Or you might just make a point of helping someone else feel better about themselves. Whichever ways you give, you'll feel so much better for having shared a part of yourself.

LESSON: By helping others, we take care of ourselves.

Giving offers us so much. It brings new experiences. It validates our existence. It provides satisfaction in our lives.

Sometimes, we readily share in the hopes that others won't have to go through the same pain we experienced during a difficult learning curve in the past. It feels good to use the insights we've gained the hard way. In the process, we learn even more about ourselves.

Other times, we give, at first, as a way to distract ourselves from painful life developments that are in the present. It's a way to feel better. Then before we know it, we're building connections to new people in a meaningful way, and doesn't that feel great?

BY HELPING OTHERS, I FOUND MYSELF
by Teri Jones

My introduction to sports was back in 1986. Through my job, I volunteered to work at a water station for the very first Los Angeles Marathon. I had no idea what a marathon was. It turned out to be fun and exciting to be around the people. The next year, I was the one doing the volunteer recruiting and I still do it 22 years later.

It wasn't until 1999, when I was 45 years old, that I ran my first marathon. I had seen a brochure about the marathon benefiting AIDS Project Los Angeles. I sent for the material and considered trying to do it. Initially, I chickened out not only because the distance was so daunting, but there was a fairly significant fundraising commitment that scared me. A few weeks later, I received a call from my friend Kathy's husband. She had asked him to call me to let me know she'd gone out of town— her 34-year-old brother had just died from AIDS. I had known

Kathy for seven years and she never mentioned a brother. Kathy would later share that she didn't approve of his lifestyle so they were estranged. After he died, she was overwhelmed with grief, sadness and guilt, learning the terrible conditions that he lived and died in. You've probably figured out what happened next. I immediately sent in my commitment form to run in the AIDS Marathon and participated in its training program. I ended up raising $5,500 in memory of Kathy's brother.

I continued doing marathons after that initial year for a couple of reasons. First was the impact it had on me and how I viewed challenges. What I got most out of completing the marathon was not that I was a jock, but that all of a sudden I realized I was capable of accomplishing anything I set my mind on doing. I learned to believe in myself, to never say "never." I developed the confidence to always go for whatever it was I wanted to do. Secondly, I wanted to share what I had learned and make it matter to more than just me. Ultimately, I completed five marathons in a four-and-a-half-year time period, all for charitable causes. I was a pace group leader or "team mentor" in all five. I had from 14 people to as many as 21 in my pace groups. I took personal responsibility for each and every person in the group. I wanted to make sure that they were successful so that they, too, could transfer the lessons learned from the discipline required to train for a marathon into their everyday lives. I knew each of them would leave a better person with endless growth potential.

Participating in my first Danskin triathlon in 2005 was another step toward accomplishing something that seemed so out of my reach. I would encourage anyone, regardless of fitness level or physique, to do the Danskin. The race is superbly organized, the participants are kind and supportive, and it will be the most exhilarating feeling you'll ever experience when you cross that finish line.

While I'll never be a world-class athlete (I think I would have had to start before I was 45), I am an athlete. In addition to the marathons, I have now completed seven triathlons, two of which were Danskins. I do want to make it clear to anyone who may think I've become a "superjock" that I don't do any of these things fast. I'm not a great swimmer. You shouldn't be surprised to see me rolled over doing the back stroke while I catch my breath and relax my arms. I will never be a speedster on the bike. Instead, I value the time it gives me to rest from the swim while seated and prepare for the run. Lastly, I take walk breaks on the run. It helps to keep me injury-free while still covering the distance. For me, it's not about my time on the event—it's all about the accomplishment.

The real reason I'm sharing my story, though, is that I want to reveal another lesson I've learned in hopes of helping others. I want to provide encouragement to all the women out there who are held back by self-doubt, low self-esteem and fear of failure.

I grew up in a very dysfunctional home. There was alcoholism, suicide, and abuse. As a result, I grew up very withdrawn and afraid and didn't trust anyone. I was a forlorn child who sat alone in the schoolyard while others played. I didn't have parental support or role models to show me how to love and nurture or to value education and exercise. I was ridiculed at school because I was a chubby kid. It drove me into a lonely, pathetic existence. I lost three mothers by the time I was 22: my birth mother to abandonment, the second to suicide when she was 36, and the third from a tragic car accident, also at the age of 36. Because of that first marathon which led to my becoming "an athlete," I turned my life around at 45 as I learned, for the first time, that I could accomplish whatever goal I set for myself. I hope someday to be in a place to help people tap into their inner soul before they allow a self-destructive state to rob them of too much of their lives. In the meantime, I hope that sharing my story might leave an impression on others so that they, too, can overcome a dysfunctional upbringing and feel good about themselves.

Remember, your limitations are the boundaries you put on yourself.

Teri Jones, 53, is the mother of one daughter. In addition to completing the marathons and triathlons as described, she has completed three bike rides down Highway One from San Francisco to Los Angeles to benefit the Arthritis Foundation for which she serves as the tour's "little mother," providing advice and encouragement to race "newbies."

MY STORY OF SURVIVAL AND HOPE
by Dessa Dzubek

I know the pain and shame of being in a domestic relationship that includes physical and verbal abuse. I had everything going for me in my professional life but my personal life was a mess. I thought to myself, "How could I have made so many good career choices and at the same time allowed myself to get into a violent domestic relationship?"

I am a 36-year-old Hispanic female with a degree in Business Management. Since graduating from college, I've worked for a Fortune 500 company for over 15 years. I have climbed the corporate ladder, having been promoted five times and winning several awards with the company.

I used to blame myself for all the difficulties in my 10-year marriage. The violent roller-coaster ride started during the first month we were married. One night, my now ex-husband, Ralph, came home late at 4 AM, completely intoxicated. He had never called to tell me he would be late and I was concerned. My questions made him extremely irritated. He then grabbed me by the neck and began choking me to shut me up. He threw the alarm clock against the wall and it shattered into pieces. He then threw me on the couch and told me "to shut the f*** up, you dumb bitch." I was scared for my life and quickly darted to the phone and dialed 911. As the operator asked, "Is this an emergency?" I said "yes." Ralph grabbed the phone and hung it up. The phone then rang and the emergency dispatcher asked again, "Is this an emergency?" Ralph said he was sorry for the call and that there was no emergency. I yelled, "Yes, it is" in the background, and within five minutes, the police were at our front door. Ralph was taken in handcuffs to the county jail and the police questioned me about his behavior. They took pictures of the red welts on my neck. The next morning, I was at the county courthouse. I saw, with embarrassment, Ralph in a blue jumpsuit with both hands cuffed behind him. In my mind, I thought, *How can this be happening to me? Wake me up. This must be a bad dream.* In front of over 50 people, the judge asked if I wanted to press charges. I said "no" to protect my husband. I just wanted to get out of there.

The same day, I spoke with Ralph's mom who was furious with me. She said, "How could you call the police? You should have just left the house. You know how he gets when he drinks." I told her he was choking me and I was scared for my life. To this day, his entire family makes excuses to mask his dependency on alcohol and the violent physical and verbal outbreaks. His sister even told me that I should have known all this before I got married—that Ralph's entire family has lots of issues.

My stories of more verbal and physical abuse with Ralph are endless. I recommended that he get alcohol counseling and marriage counseling but he told me, "Why, so they can point out what's wrong with me and you can laugh at me?" He never went for counseling and I continued to make excuses for his actions. Through all of this, I became dependent on antidepressants, sleeping pills, and alcohol. I suffered a nervous breakdown and finally realized it was time to get help for myself after I considered suicide. I did not want to give up on life and me. I recognized that if I had taken my own life, Ralph would have won. I got the help I needed through family and friends and realized I needed positive outlets.

I decided to train for a triathlon as a way to set a positive goal and beneficial focus. I remember, at one time when I was thinking about doing a Danskin race, my then-husband said, "What do you want to prove?" He would always deter me from my personal goals. My journey of survival and hope has allowed me to drive negative thoughts like these from my head and focus on the positive. I recovered from my alcohol and antidepressant addictions, learned how to eat healthy, and became more fit and confident. I trained vigorously for the swim, bike, and run.

I was very proud when I completed my first triathlon. I am now training for a half marathon. I am so happy with myself but it has taken a lot of personal work and soul-searching. I have several other things to accomplish in this beautiful life I now have.

I want to help others by becoming an advocate for women suffering from domestic violence and sharing what I've learned and overcome. I now know that a victim can become VICTORIOUS in life by lifting herself out of the negative situation she is involved in. A healing process must take place inside and she can't be afraid to ask for help. The support allows her to rebuild her foundation and live life freely from the shackles that once bound her. I know the pain and shame associated with being in a domestic relationship of physical and verbal abuse. I was embarrassed and ashamed to tell others. I share my story, knowing I can lead the way for other women who suffer from abuse and violence.

There's a quote from Lance Armstrong I love, about needing to go all the way when you get a second chance in life. This is what I plan on doing.

Dessa Dzubek endured a long and painful divorce, giving up her home, two cars, a Harley motorcycle, and half her retirement money in the process. As she says, "I had to accept those were only material items. I can rebuild my life and I'm so happy to have my second chance."

When we reach out and give to others, we never know where that step might lead. At one time, I left the nine-to-five (or was it eight-to-eight?) business world, and was adjusting to working in my family business. I joined a wonderful women's networking group, the UCWBG, which is affiliated with the university where I got my MBA, and I volunteered soon afterwards to serve on the group's board (staying for five years including a year as president!). I learned so much from those women, about business and life, and gained many friends. For instance, one of the women told me about a book which was very helpful in my journey of recovery from the kidney issues that I previously described. (Thanks, Dubravka!) My initial impulse to connect by volunteering my time led to so much more than I ever imagined.

As you read in the first story above, the last 20 years of Teri's adult life are characterized by volunteerism and giving to others. When she was in her 30s, working the water station at the LA Marathon provided a new purpose in Teri's life. Through her volunteer efforts, Teri began to create a sense of connection and community that was missing during her isolated and lonely childhood.

Later, in an effort to support her friend Kathy (who had lost a brother to AIDS), Teri ran her first marathon. Of course, Teri reaped rewards of her own, even though her motivation was to do something for another by raising money to benefit AIDS research. In training for the marathon, she became more physically fit. As a result of her physical activity, Teri gained psychological benefits including an improved outlook and sense of optimism. This was a major turning point in Teri's life as she realized she could accomplish whatever she set her mind on doing—she didn't have to spend her life in a state of hopelessness and despair, brought on by the injustices of her childhood.

With such strong rewards for her volunteer efforts, Teri decided to devote her life to helping others by being a mentor and role model. And she readily shares the story of her painful past in an effort to help others who can relate to her experience.

Dessa's story shares many of the same characteristics of Teri's. She, too, shares her painful past, involving spousal abuse and violence in her case, to offer hope and encouragement to others in similar positions. Dessa describes the shame she felt as well as how she made excuses for her abusive then-husband for 10 years, knowing others face similar challenges now. Like Teri, Dessa aspires to serve as a role model to demonstrate that it's possible to move on and live a new and better life. By sharing her lessons learned, she's creating something positive out of a rough past situation.

LESSON: By giving to others, you realize the purpose of your unique knowledge, gifts, and skills.

Caring comes naturally to human beings. So if we can find a way to share our knowledge, gifts and skills during a difficult time, then we can find purpose during a challenge.

FROM THE OTHER SIDE OF THE FINISH LINE
by Ruth Kaminski

After completing my first Danskin and another triathlon that same year, I was excited to see what I could accomplish during the next triathlon season. Unfortunately, very early in the season, I became injured and was unable to compete in *even one* event!

I spoke of my disappointment with Sally Edwards at one of the Danskin training seminars, and she promptly told me that I needed to be a Danskin Swim Angel. I was so excited at the prospect and eagerly sent off a request. My excitement came to a screeching halt when I was informed that the Swim Angel program (one of the most popular volunteer positions) was filled and had a wait list. Almost in tears, I emailed Sally of my (well, at least in my mind) "tragedy." Sally promptly offered to let me be her assistant the day of the race. I was thrilled to be involved in any way possible since my daughter would be completing her first triathlon that day. I also had several friends competing—some for the first time, others seasoned triathletes.

I was blessed to be out on the dock beside Sally. I stood there with Sally, holding her megaphone and the monkey balloon that was a symbol of the fears the women needed to let go. I cheered myself hoarse as I watched 38 waves of women step into the water to begin the race. I looked out at those women and saw their fear and anxiety, the nervous tension. I watched Sally project her courage, her heart, her belief in each one of them out over them like a warm blanket to take away the chill of the lake. Sally provided courage and strength for those that were, at that moment, having a hard time drawing on their inner athlete.

After starting the waves, Sally headed out to swim with the (would be) final swimmer. I moved over to the area in which the swimmers were exiting the lake. I saw a much different look on those faces. I saw confidence in what they had just tackled; I saw smiles as they were cheered on by the crowd, and I saw a lot of relief to have one of the events behind them. When Sally came up with the next-to-last swimmer, the roar of the crowd was deafening. The Swim Angels gathered and created a swim noodle arch for this swimmer to pass under. The rest of the volunteers were high-fiving her and telling her how great she did. She was out of breath but smiling. The most touching moment came when Sally put her arm around that swimmer's shoulders and turned her toward the water. Sally pointed to the first marker, then the second, then the place she had just exited the water. Finally, Sally looked her in the eye and simply said: "Look what you just did. You CAN do this triathlon!" That was all it took: that final swimmer took off up the chute to the transition area, ready to tackle the bike.

The day wore on, and we were at the finish line congratulating athletes as they came in. There I got to spend some time with Sally Edwards, Maggie Sullivan (the Danskin Women's Triathlon Series Director), and Ardis Bow (coordinator of the Swim Angel program). I discovered that Sally, Maggie and Ardis are truly there for the athletes. These three caring, loving women wholeheartedly want to empower those women who put themselves to the test in doing an endurance event. Repeatedly, I was amazed by the encouragement, concern and care they exhibited. They tirelessly gave the same level of enthusiasm and respect to each woman who came across that line. What amazing hearts and souls those women have!

Finally, Sally took off to run the last couple of miles with the athlete who would have been the final finisher, if not for Sally. Only about 100 or so spectators were left; it had been over six hours since the start of the race. I was worried that there would not be enough fanfare to herald this brave woman in. I needn't have worried. Those 100 people sounded like a thousand as Sally, the Team Danskin Training Coaches and Workout Leaders, and that woman athlete came into sight, working their way to the finish line. All the volunteers were clapping and cheering and screaming encouragement as she crossed that finish line. I was not the only one with tears of joy streaming down my face. As the finisher Sally had accompanied stopped to catch her breath, Sally gave her a hug and then stepped back to allow the rest of us to get in there and share congratulatory hugs. This woman obviously had struggled, but did not give up. In that moment, I realized just why Sally, Maggie and Ardis are so committed to this endeavor. When you are able to stand in the presence of someone who has accomplished the seemingly unattainable, it humbles you—it changes you even more than when you crossed the finish line yourself. The inspiration that woman provided will always be with me.

Being on the "other side" of the finish line was such an incredible day for me. I got to see my daughter start the swim and run portions. I was there to hug her immediately after she crossed the finish line. I got to look into the beaming, sweaty, tired face of that woman Sally had accompanied over the finish line—a woman who had so much courage, so much heart and strength. I was changed in a way that I never would have been if I had been able to participate as an athlete. Eleanor Roosevelt said, "You gain strength, courage and confidence by every experience in which you really stop to look fear in the face. You must do the thing you think you cannot do."

Ruth Kaminski completed her first triathlon at the age of 50, as included in Chapter 2. Due to an injury that prevented her from training, she returned to the Danskin triathlon in Seattle the following year, as a volunteer.

FILLING THE VOID
by Mona Frisbie

It wasn't until I was out of college, in my 20s, that I became hooked on running. This happened after I started running with a friend. I trained six days per week and felt better than ever. People commented how terrific I looked since I started running (and shed the extra pounds from college). I became really good at running and it felt so natural. I competed in local 5k road races, 10ks, and eventually half marathons—finishing every race feeling stronger and stronger and reaching personal bests. Running became my constitution. Everyone knew me as "the runner." I eventually trained 70 miles per week and ran the Chicago Marathon in the early 1980s. What a great feeling of accomplishment! I signed up the next year and ran the marathon once again. I ran through my 20s and 30s.

After all the years of running, my body started to break down. My knees could not take all the miles, so I started cross-training. I joined the local YMCA and started to swim five days per week. As a result, I became a strong swimmer. I tried running again after my son was born. My body just couldn't take all the pounding anymore so I started to cut back on the miles.

A dear friend from the YMCA talked me into signing up for the Chicago Triathlon. I couldn't resist. I already had the swimming and running down. I just had to work on my biking skills. In 1999, I finished the Chicago Triathlon strong. I was addicted. I had triathlon fever and signed up for the next year's event. I loved the cross-training and felt stronger than I had ever been. It was such a high competing in triathlons and I managed to finish fourth place in my age group. My two children would come watch me compete. It was one of the best times of my life to have them see me do something I loved so much and worked so hard to accomplish.

A number of years later, I developed a serious running injury that required me to stop running altogether. I was devastated. Running was such a big part of who I was—how could I give this up? I had dreams of triathlons to compete in, races to run, and personal records to beat. After running for 25 years, my life changed so quickly. I realized I had to fill a huge void and reinvent myself. But with what?

A friend from my YMCA spin class invited me to become a Team Danskin Training Workout Leader for a group of women training for their first triathlon. I hesitated to join because I wasn't sure I had anything to contribute. A little voice inside my head said, "Just do it." I couldn't participate in a triathlon again but I could certainly help others achieve their dreams and goals of finishing their first triathlon. I realized that this opportunity could be a wonderful way for me to fill my void.

In the spring of 2007, I first met the women on the training team. Every woman had her own story to share and this incredible determination to finish a triathlon. I really enjoyed the twice-a-week group training sessions and found myself looking forward to the next meeting. The team members were remarkable. I was able to inspire some of them, motivate others to do an extra lap, laugh with them through a hard workout, and carry water bottles for them on their run. In the end, I actually felt like I had something to offer. They asked for my advice on triathlon transitions, and listened to what I had to share with them. This was such a positive experience for me: I had no idea I would get so much out of this personally. I have the team coaches, Susan Kane and Jean Spiegelhalter, to thank for helping me discover the next phase of my life as a non-running athlete.

After years of competing as a top-finishing age grouper in marathons and triathlons, Mona Frisbie joined the Chicago Northwest

Suburbs Team Danskin Training as a Workout Leader. She is the mother of two children. With her husband, she founded a grassroots health initiative to help consumers make informed decisions about their healthcare spending, www.outofpocket.com.

In sharing our strengths, we touch another life, and help someone else grow. Along the way, we learn from those we support. Helping others also provides perspective. There's always someone who is dealing with a bigger challenge than we are.

Both Mona and Ruth had experienced the joy and personal empowerment that came from their athletic endeavors. Physical fitness became an important and integral part of each of their lives. When injuries forced them to put their respective passions on hold, their reactions were to find ways to impart what they had learned with others, to share their insights. These two women ended up being inspired by those they were helping.

Ruth also received a great deal of inspiration by watching the leaders of the Danskin Women's Triathlon Series—Sally, Maggie and Ardis—women who put their hearts into their roles with the event. Ruth was truly inspired by the compassion she saw each of these women share with the thousands of participants.

LESSON: Giving is easy when supporting a cause you believe in.

There are an almost limitless number of causes you can support. Whatever your cause, make a difference in a way that makes sense in your life today. At various points, how you're best able to contribute may change. When you have the time, volunteer to support an activity of the cause you believe in. Financial support is always needed and welcome, too, of course. In fact, a recent study covered in the journal

Science found that the biggest givers of donations to causes and gifts to others were happier than people who spent more of their own money on themselves.[11]

SUPPORTING AN IMPORTANT CAUSE
by Darlene Nelson-Watkins

An important reason why I participated in the Danskin race was helping to raise funds to fight cancer and to see all those survivors in the race. That was uplifting to me.

Crossing the finish line meant I finished what I set out to do, including helping to fight cancer. The disease of cancer does not discriminate who it affects. My sister, brother and I come from parents of different races. Our parents are from Norway. Our mother is black. She is a survivor of breast cancer. Our father is white. He had prostate cancer. I don't take for granted how seriously this disease can affect a person.

I used to think that as long as cancer was identified early enough and you got treatment, you'd have a good chance of survival. I since have learned what a person has to go through during the crisis. Participating in the Danskin race was a way for me to support cancer research and give back in the fight of this terrible disease.

Darlene Nelson-Watkins is a member of Team Dream. She is the mother of a son, Jason.

It's easiest to support a cause that we can relate to personally—that we have some sort of connection with.

For many women who consider the Danskin triathlon, the event's contribution to breast cancer research is the final tipping point for getting involved. Darlene of Team Dream felt that way.

This certainly was also the case in my own decision when I contemplated my first Danskin triathlon. I lost a grandmother I never knew to breast cancer. She died while my mom was still in high school. I also have a good friend and mentor from my early career days, Kathy, who has battled breast cancer since 1993. My cousin, Mary, continues to fight a valiant struggle against Stage IV breast cancer. Two other friends from a group of neighborhood moms are now cancer-free after their own series of treatments. So, supporting breast cancer research is a cause that's important to me.

What cause calls to you? If you're seeking an athletic challenge, consider a triathlon, 10k, 5k or other sports-centered event that supports it.

LESSON: You may never know the impact of a little act of kindness.

Sometimes it's the little things that make a big difference. Sharing a smile or a compliment with a stranger can make their day. Simple acts of kindness make a positive difference in the world, one small act at a time.

AN ANGEL TO ME
by Brenda Umbrianna

There I was, at the start of the Webster Danskin race. I had trained hard, had worked hard and I was ready... or so I thought. I was standing in the water, repeating my mantra, "I am a fantastic swimmer." This was my first triathlon and I was ready to pull off some great times. That was the reason for participating: to reach my goals and gain some experience for the next race. As I started the swim leg, my confidence plummeted. I suddenly felt restricted and breathing became difficult. I thought I would have to end my race right there in the water.

The woman swimming beside me must have noticed my erratic strokes and the panic on my face. She asked if I was okay. When I said "No," she stopped racing and swam over to me. She was not a Swim Angel, but she was an angel to me. She held on to my hand and raised her other hand to call for a kayak. I did not have my wits about me to call for help on my own. This woman stayed with me until I had rested and caught my breath. As I watched her swim away, it became clear to me why I had signed on for this challenge. Instantly, race times and competitors did not matter. I was surrounded by all these wonderful, powerful, supportive women. From that moment on, I enjoyed the journey.

I made it a point to compliment and encourage every woman I saw, especially those who were struggling. I am not the same woman who started the race and I am glad I had the opportunity to discover my inner athlete and appreciate the beauty and strength in my fellow sisters. I hope to be able to thank my angel personally when I return to the Danskin next year.

Brenda Umbrianna, 36, completed her first Danskin Triathlon in 2005. She is married and the mother of Andrew (7) and Delaney (5). She is a stay-at-home mom working towards a Masters Degree in Early Childhood Education and is currently a Workout Leader for Metro-South Boston Danskin Women's Triathlon Team. In addition to spending time with her family, she enjoys reading, yoga, and working in her garden.

It costs us nothing to share a smile or an encouraging word. Being kind can be as simple as holding the door open for the next person or letting another car merge in front of you with a friendly wave.

Brenda's story illustrates the power of a simple act of kindness. An unnamed woman stopped to help as Brenda panicked on her swim during the Danskin triathlon. This "good Samaritan" calmed Brenda while calling for help from the life guards. This may have been an effort the other woman put forth without a second thought. Yet her kindness meant the world to Brenda. Once Brenda regained her confidence for the swim, she changed her entire attitude about finishing the race. The event was no longer about the time she took to complete it. Being a part of the Danskin became about offering support to other women like she had received from her personal swim angel.

Go ahead. Make someone's day! How can you make a small difference in another life today by being kind?

LESSON: Be a mentor or a role model.

In Chapter 8, I discussed the need to build your team and get support for accomplishing your goals and living an authentic life. Sometimes that means building a team made of friends and/or family. Other times that involves hiring a coach to mentor and advise you through the process. Now we look at the opposite side of that equation—being a mentor or role model yourself.

YOU DON'T ALWAYS HAVE TO LEARN IT THE HARD WAY
by Susan Farago

I have looked into the eyes of Danskin athletes and seen the excitement and passion of doing something for themselves— perhaps for the first time in a long time OR (even more horrifying) for the first time *ever*. I decided I wanted to give back to the sport of triathlon, and more specifically, to women in the sport.

I was asked to be a Team Danskin Training Workout Leader in 2003, which led to my being a Team Danskin assistant coach in 2004 and 2006. I had learned things the hard way training for my first Danskin triathlon and I wanted to share my "what not to do" experiences with other women so they wouldn't have to go through the same lessons unnecessarily. Additionally, showing them how to change a tire wasn't only about changing a tire, but rather it was a lesson on self-reliance and empowerment. Explaining to them how to fuel for training and racing wasn't about the latest diet trends and fads; it was about eating smarter and educating them about what their bodies would need. A willingness to share and laugh at ourselves prompted many of the women to open up their souls for all to see—their fears, apprehensions, and self-doubts. I encouraged them to let go of these things and replace them with confidence, strength, and self-assurance… as if triathlon was some type of religion that would save their souls. For some, it was.

Susan Farago is from Austin, Texas. Her story in Chapter 4 describes her triathlon experiences ranging from the Danskin to the Ironman Hawaii World Championship.

ONE GESTURE AT A TIME
by Janice Cohen

As the assistant coach for the Connecticut Heart Zones Team Danskin Training, I have enjoyed every second of our eight-week training. Working with the "Tri-Ladies," as we affectionately called them, was a labor of love! Training and motivating a diverse group of women, ranging in age from 20 to 63 meant more to me than any event I have done individually. The whole (our group of Tri-Ladies) was definitely greater than the sum of its parts, which made this yet another peak Danskin experience for me.

To quote an email from one of our team members: "I hope you understand the power of your positivity and nurturance. I am a big believer in the power of change, one gesture at a time. Your influence impacted me and I went back to the world uplifted and, hopefully, passed some of that positivity on to the next and on and on. It's great stuff."

I couldn't have said it better!

Janice Cohen shared this observation after her experience as an assistant coach for Team Danskin training.

Do you recall Teri's and Dessa's stories from the beginning of this chapter? Both of those women viewed becoming a role model to others as helpful in overcoming a life challenge. All of these women—Teri, Dessa, Susan and Janice—have been rewarded when sharing their experiences and serving as role models to other women.

Susan's story talks about the power of coaching other women to get ready for their first triathlons. Even though Susan had immense demands on her time between her job and her own training (including training for Ironman competitions), she found great rewards in taking the time to be a mentor to Danskin women. It provided the opportunity to share what she had learned the hard way and to give back to the sport that had provided so much to her.

As an assistant coach for Team Danskin Training in Connecticut, Janice was a role model to the varied members of her team. In return, she experienced the gratitude for the impact she had made on her team members' lives. Working with the group proved to be a powerful, synergistic experience with the "whole being greater than the sum of its parts."

Why not consider becoming a mentor or a role model, too? It's an opportunity to share what you've learned over the course of your life.

Share the "what NOT to do" lessons from what you've experienced as well as your positive insights.

> **NOTE:** In considering mentoring or becoming a role model, it's important to be selective about what you choose and the depth of your commitment. As was discussed earlier in the book, women can have a tendency to give too much. There's a fine line between making a difference and taking on more than is good for you. Keep this in mind as you take on leadership roles.

LESSON: Give as you receive.

Use the energy you gain from the kindness of others to give back to someone else. Whether that's a kind word of encouragement to another person, or volunteering to work for a good cause, share what you have to offer with someone else. Remember that you also had help along the way.

THE GOLDEN RULE
by Susan Denini

The Danskin race day is something you just have to experience. The enormous sea of bikes racked up in rows is truly a sight to behold, as is the incredible number of amazing women of all shapes, sizes and ages—all ready to take on the challenge! All the participants had facial expressions that combined excitement, fear, exhilaration, astonishment and determination. I went through every one of those expressions and a few more myself!

I felt very lucky and, even more, touched and appreciative to have my family and so many friends come out to cheer me on. They had signs and balloons and cheered so loudly that it was hard not to break into tears each time I saw them. And it wasn't just the people I knew. The overwhelming positive support and affirmations from everyone participating and watching was contagious. You couldn't be there and not catch it!

And the volunteers! Don't even get me started on the volunteers! I cannot believe the sheer number of incredible people who run and organize this event. And it wouldn't happen without the volunteers. They were nothing but smiles from the very beginning. Even on the registration day, I met some women who were so excited that it was my first time and were full of little tidbits of advice… "Get some Gatorade and the blue is the best!" "Bring some extra water that you can pour over your feet to wash them off after the swim." "Unroll your socks and put them in your shoes for the transition—every second counts." There are memories of so many volunteers that run through my head when I think back, but here are some I'd like to mention:

- The man who wrote my race number on my arms and legs and said, "Good luck, you're gonna do great!"

- The girl who gave me my race shirt and asked if I was sure I needed the 2X size. (Bless her heart!)

- The guy in the kayak who came after me as I swam farther and farther off course toward the middle of the lake on the swim. "You're doing great," he said. "Just get back on course!"

- All the wonderful people encouraging us on the bike ride as we tried to maneuver that nasty steep curve to get onto the bridge. (I made it!)

- The lone volunteers sitting out in the middle of the I-90 bridge in the scorching sun yelling, "You're doing great" at every bike that whizzed past them.

- The "bike guys" who pumped my front tire up before the race AND at the turnaround on the bridge. (Stupid dang tire!)

- The little boy who was so excited to douse me with a cup of water on the run. (At least he asked first!)

- The woman at the 2-mile marker on the run who I just had to stop and hug for her endless enthusiasm.

- The volunteer who gave me a huge hug and whispered, "You are incredible" in my ear at the end of the race.

- The great people who were cutting up oranges and spreading our choice of peanut butter or cream cheese on bagels in the after-race booths.

I have great memories and many wonderful stories I could share from this experience, but one of my favorites took place very close to the end of the race. About 2.5 miles into the run, there was a hill. Really just one extra-long block, it had a significant incline which wasn't easy to take. Thankfully, there were lots of encouraging fans along the sidewalks and a great group of guys on drums banging out a tune with the perfect rhythm to help you hoof your way up.

As I was approaching the hill, I met this wonderful older woman. I laughed at how great the drummers were and she agreed, but commented that she would be walking to the beat and not running up the hill. I assured her that I wasn't going to run either and was happy to walk along with her. The woman said that she might go too slowly for me and expressed doubt about making it at all. I told her that was nonsense! We were within a half mile of the finish line—she had already done it! The lady then explained that she had severe arthritis in her feet and had decided to do the Danskin as an accomplishment to look back on when she could no longer walk at all. I was moved by her story of determination and quickly shared my story with her.

We congratulated each other and started up the hill together in step with the drumming but realized all too soon what a quick pace it was. She started to slow down a bit and told me again that she didn't think she could make it. I took her hand in mine and pulled her close to my side. I said we'd take shorter steps together but we'd stay in rhythm. About halfway up, she let out a big sigh and started to shake her head. I told her not to look up but just to concentrate on the step in front of us and breathe to the rhythm. Before either of us knew it, we were at the top. We had really pushed and my legs were burning and I know she was feeling the heat as well. We were both out of breath, smiling and crying. She squeezed my hand tightly and said, "Thank you!" I squeezed back and said, "You're amazing." There just weren't any more words we could share that could express what we were both feeling. We walked a bit further, hand in hand. Then I told her that I was going to start running again at the end of the block. She squeezed my hand again and blew me a kiss. I didn't catch her name but her story is part of mine forever!

As I approached the finish line, my ears were ringing. I could hear everyone cheering and clapping along the side-lines, however all I could concentrate on was my own breathing as I tried desperately not to start bawling! The gravity of all I had done in the last year and a half was hitting me and my head was spinning. My legs were burning again but I was determined to RUN across the finish line. I did—and I am not the same woman I was when I started. Now I know I can do anything I put my mind on doing.

Susan Denini completed her first Danskin after losing over 125 pounds. More of her story is included in Chapter 6.

Find a way to invest some of your energy back into our world. As you receive energy from the support of others, pass it on. You will be repaid many times in return.

Completing her first triathlon was a powerful milestone for Susan, who was celebrating her substantial weight-loss and a new focus on fitness and taking care of herself. Crossing the finish line was a momentous experience for her. Yet of all the feelings and thoughts she had, it is the efforts of all the volunteers who supported the race that came up first in her recollections of the day. In spite of all the energy that completing her first race required, Susan was able to be there for another woman who faced her own daunting challenge at the Danskin in the form of arthritis. In giving to this other woman, Susan created a memorable moment and supplied needed support. She gave back in the midst of receiving so much from others herself.

Pay It Forward

You can make the world a better place, just like all the volunteers at the Danskin races and other triathlon events. As others have helped you along the way in life, "pay it forward" to someone else. It doesn't have to be about an earth-shattering change. Even one small gesture at a time makes a difference. Isn't connecting with others what life is all about?

Consider all the women who readily shared their stories for this book. Not even one asked for compensation. Stories came from busy women who had to make an effort to find the time to document their experiences. The amazing women who shared their stories wanted to share what they had learned in hopes of helping someone else.

Finding the time to give to others or to volunteer to a worthy cause often isn't easy for most of us. But you can do it. Perform acts of kindness or generosity just because it will make YOU feel better.

When volunteering for a cause, pick one you're most passionate about or have some personal connection with—this will make it that much easier to find the energy and the time. There are a seemingly infinite number of causes to support. Make your choice, and contribute in whatever way is appropriate for you at this time in your life.

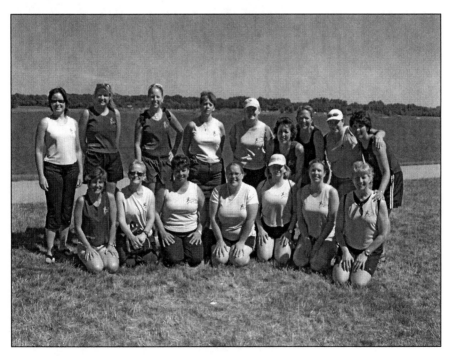

2007 TEAM DANSKIN TRAINING CHICAGO NW SUBURBS, INCLUDING COACHES AND WORKOUT LEADERS

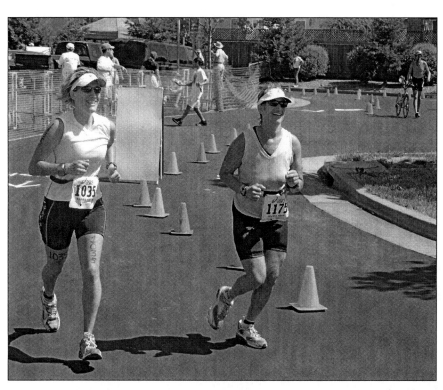

Pamela Kropf (on left) and friend, ready to
fly over the finish line together

CHAPTER 10

Now Take Flight!

Sharing our stories has long been a powerful tool for women as we attempt to transform ourselves and soar into our futures. Hearing or reading the words of other women, and witnessing their journeys, gives us a new glimpse of our own possibilities. We begin to understand that if something is possible for another—such as flying over a triathlon's finish line—then it can also be possible *for us*. We get ideas for handling challenges. We see new ways of being that are more satisfying. We learn that we can accomplish whatever we set our minds to do.

Our days are full of choices. It's up to you to make the choices that will bring the most joy and happiness into your life… to create a life that is consistent with your beliefs and values… a life that is true to who you are… a self-satisfying, authentic and empowered life.

What Brings Us Happiness?

According to *Pursuit of Happiness* author David G. Meyers, PhD, happiness is NOT tied to age, wealth, sex, level of education, race, the size of the house we live in, or the kind of car we drive. Factors that DO contribute to happiness include:

- Fit and healthy bodies
- Realistic goals and expectations

- Positive self-esteem
- Feelings of control
- Optimism
- Outgoingness
- Supportive friendships
- A socially intimate, sexually warm, equitable marriage
- Challenging work and active leisure
- Faith that encompasses communal support, purpose, acceptance, outward focus, and hope.

Note that physical fitness and health are at the top of the list to keys to happiness!

Participation in triathlons can contribute positively to many of the other factors on this list in addition to the first one. With proper training, completing a triathlon can provide a realistic goal and is a form of active leisure. Triathlon training can produce positive self-esteem and feelings of control and optimism. In how many stories did we hear, "I learned that if I could complete this triathlon, I could accomplish anything I set my mind on doing"? Plus success for many of the triathletes was influenced by the support of friends, family members, or a training team or coach. Given all the benefits that contribute to happiness, it's no wonder that the number of women who participate in triathlons is growing!

Your Transition to New Athletic Achievement

Have you been inspired to move forward with a new fitness goal as the result of reading this book? A triathlon, 5k, 10k, or even an aquabike or duathlon? Once you start training, slowly but surely, you'll begin to see some progress. Signs will emerge which show that you are empowering your inner athlete. You'll realize that your muscles are sore because you're using them in a new way—and that's a good thing. You'll experience feelings of confidence that come with sports training. You'll begin to change. Your transition to a more fit human being has begun!

For those who have chosen triathlon as their goal, I highly recommend Sally Edwards' books, *Triathlons for Women* or *The Complete Book of Triathlons* for help with developing your plan.

Have a Plan, and Work It!

That's right... once you've identified a goal that brings you happiness and is true to who you are, you'll need to develop a plan and begin to implement it.

But before we can prepare a plan to achieve our goal, we must understand our starting point—who we are and where we are. Our starting point is so influenced by our life experiences: both the facts of our lives and the interpretation we put on those facts. By objectively separating fact from interpretation, we can identify the strengths which are transferable to other aspects of our lives. We also need to let go of the self-limiting beliefs of our old story so we are unencumbered as we proceed on our journey.

Later, working the plan will mean traveling from where you are to where you want to be. It will require that you let go of past ways of thinking and doing things to move on to something new and better.

In setting your goal, and in designing the plan to achieve your goal, follow your heart. Your brain may give you all kinds of conflicting messages. You won't go wrong if you act based on desire and passion driven by your heart.

(For more on goals, go back to Chapter 5.)

Transition Lessons from Within the Triathlon Itself

Throughout the stories in this book, lessons learned through triathlon experiences have been applied to other aspects of women's lives. In the same way, transitions which occur at two points *during* an actual triathlon can teach us. Although transitions are an expected part of the race, as in life, they can present new challenges for us.

First, as we get *out of the water from our swim* (Success #1!), having been horizontal and buoyant for 15 to 30 minutes or more, a change is thrust upon us as we put weight on our legs. We run to the transition area where we must find our bike and gear amongst the equipment of thousands of other triathletes. We deal with the discomfort of getting the sand or dirt off our feet. We need to go from wet to dry enough to put on our socks (maybe), bike shoes, helmets. We're forced to walk to the bike start on legs that are still wobbly from the swim. As triathletes, we have no choice but to continue through the transition in order to proceed from the swim to the bike. And then we head off on a bike path of, say, 12 miles. It's likely to be fairly unfamiliar territory because the bike route is so much longer than the swimming course. In the lake, it's easy to see the route from start to finish. But what's coming up next on the bike path? Curves? Hills? Bumpy pavement? An unanticipated long line of participants you hope to pass on the course?

Then, in a blur, we complete our bike ride (Success #2!), and once again find ourselves in the midst of a transition. This second one is a much more challenging transition: *Going from the bike to the run.* We rack our bikes, take off our helmets, perhaps change our shoes and throw on a visor. And we're ready to head off on the final part of this journey. But this transition is tough. Getting our legs to walk or run after biking 45 minutes or more is not easy. Our muscles contract. At first, every step is a challenge. Every step completed becomes an accomplishment. Slowly but surely, we regain our footing. Eventually we realize that the transition is behind us. The goal, flying over the finish line, is now in sight. We can achieve it!

Life Transitions: What to Expect

The experience of triathlon course-transitions provides a model we all can apply to the transitions in our lives. We see that the discomfort of a transition gives way to an accomplishment, and that we must persevere. A wiser, more fulfilled life awaits our new beginning.

Like the transition to fit triathlete, there are many other kinds of transitions in life that are positive and voluntary—where we intentionally work the plan to get to a better place. For instance, transitions may be due to:

- Leaving for college
- Giving birth to a child
- Relocating
- Getting married
- Starting a new job

Other transitions may be thrust upon us when we least expect them. Life transitions for which we have no choice include:

- Accidents
- Serious illnesses
- Being fired or laid off from a job
- Death of a loved one
- An unexpected divorce

The first step in successfully dealing with transitions is awareness—knowing that you are in the midst of a period of change and a time of uncertainty. Expect that during this time, you will feel uncomfortable. Inevitably, self-doubt will rear its head to entice you to go back to the old way because it seems easier than the uncertainty that is inescapable in a transition. "But if we let the voices of fear and doubt override what we know to be true in our heart," cautions life coach Mary Ann Bailey, "we could make decisions about our future that may not serve us well in the long run."[12]

Bailey, a Seattle, Washington life coach, specializes in helping women move through change in midlife. She describes a transition in this way:

"I compare going through a life transition to setting sail on a foggy sea. As you begin your transition, you can still see the shoreline. At this point, you may not even realize you are in a transition. You are very excited about the possibilities of changing a part of your life; and you can hardly wait to set sail and explore the distant shores.

"Yet, as you sail further out to sea, or further into your transition, you lose sight of the familiar shoreline. The fog begins to settle in around you. You can't make out where you're going, and you can no longer see where you came from.

"This feeling of drifting at sea with no port in sight can be very unnerving for many of us. We live in a culture that wants fast and definitive answers to our questions. We want quick solutions to our problems. And we want fast and easy ways out of the fog of transition...

"We need to believe that if we keep ourselves open to the experience, and if we continue to move slowly toward our goal, we will eventually sail out of the fog and find ourselves in a new and wonderful place."[13]

Despite the promise of a better way, transitions are difficult because they involve change. It can seem easier at times for us to cling to the old ways than to let go of the past and find a new way—especially when the new way involves uncertainty. To keep moving forward during a transition, we need to have a clear vision of where we want to go and who we want to be when we get there. We need to understand that the journey of transition will bring us new wisdom.

Transitions that occur as we work our plan, though uncomfortable, offer the opportunity to once again reassess who we are, what's important to us, and what our dreams and desires are.

Getting There with a Little Help

An important key to success in a time of transition is to have an appropriate support network in place. That support may come from a friend, mentor, professional coach, therapist or a combination of these sources. It may also come from a support group with similar goals. It's important to know that those around you, those closest to you, such as a parent or spouse, may not be the best source of support during your transition. As you question what is important to you for the future, you may threaten relationships with those you love.

As you change, you are changing those existing relationships. Those around you may be more comfortable with the status quo than with moving into unfamiliar territory because of your growth. If you experience resistance, remind yourself that moving to a place that's best for you in this new phase will be worth persisting—even if difficult at times.

Some of those older relationships will survive a major transition, while others won't. Meanwhile you'll be aware of the need to create additional support for the changes you're going through. In this way, people will be there to provide a forum for problem-solving, solutions and sharing.

Although your fears—the monkeys on your back—may threaten to keep you stuck, you must overcome your fears to move forward to a better place. Your connections—new and old—can provide support as you take necessary new risks in your life. If you don't take a chance and take risks that move you out of your comfort zones, you'll hazard not moving forward in your life. You may become stagnant and complacent.

Gather support for your goal, and start moving forward!

(You'll find more on building a support team in Chapter 8.)

Flying Lessons for Life

In preparing to achieve our goal of crossing the finish line—be it that of a triathlon or whatever stretch goal we set for ourselves—we begin a journey of self-discovery. We find our strengths and acknowledge our weaknesses. We detect attributes we never knew existed in our being. We learn about determination and strength of mind. We become adaptable as we adjust to the inevitable roadblocks and complications that occur on our journey.

As women, we are pulled in a multitude of directions, trying to take care of everyone and everything in our lives. Family, career, friends—too often we neglect to make time for ourselves. We may even lose sight of who we are. But by setting a personal goal, committing to it, and working toward it, we create new, positive energy that overflows into all other aspects of our life.

Setting a goal provides new inspiration and motivation. It is a means of revitalizing our existence. Each day, we wake up with a sense of purpose and vigor. It propels us forward on our journey to a place where we maximize our potential and best use our gifts. Meanwhile, how we define success and happiness must be based on our own personal definition—not someone else's solution.

In taking risks, inevitably, we will sometimes fail to achieve our intended goals. That is okay and is actually to be expected. As we look for the silver lining in the cloud of "failure," we'll find that we have learned something new while taking the risk. We have moved forward along the journey. We have increased the possibility of success the next time.

When we do succeed at achieving our goals, we'll savor the victory—even more if we had to overcome obstacles and defeats along the way. We will embrace our success and learn from it—knowing we are empowered further to take on the next goal—whatever that might be.

Take Flight!

With your new awareness of the need to take risks, to continually stretch yourself, and to redefine who you are, now is the time to take flight. The key to success is to take what you've learned in this book and put it into action. Identify a new goal. Create a plan to achieve the goal. Find a friend or support group to share the journey with. The choices are limitless. Make the choices that keep you happy and healthy. Believe in yourself and your abilities.

When we draw upon and use the power within ourselves to learn, accomplish new goals, and achieve success (*however* that success is personally defined, remember), we get a taste of personal empowerment. We see that we can make change happen in our lives. So keep moving forward to become all that you were meant to be, using your unique talents and gifts, while making a commitment to yourself to do your best. Learn to soar and take flight!

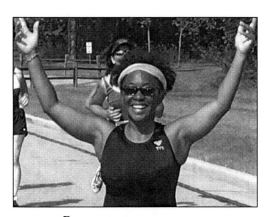

READY TO TAKE FLIGHT

Endnotes

[1] www.ironman.com/history.

[2] USA Triathlon., www.usatriathlon.org.

[3] Tim Yount, USAT, email message to author, February 27, 2008.

[4] Ibid.

[5] www.tricalifornia.com/index.cfm/sponsor_information.htm.

[6] Derrick Q. Milligan, Team Dream, http://www.teamdream.org/multisport_tidbits.php.

[7] Carol Hochman, Danskin CEO, Welcome letter, Danskin Women's Triathlon Series 2006 Program.

[8] *Health in a Heartbeat*, Dan Rudd, PhD, and Sally Edwards, MA, MBA, Heart Zones Publishing, p. 8.

[9] http://www.adventure-marathon.com/LaSalle-Bank-Chicago-Marathon-2008.aspx.

[10] Leblanc, Pamela, "Listening to her inner athlete," Cox News Service, June 5, 2005.

[11] *Science*, March 21, 2008, vol. 319: pp. 1687-1688.

[12] Bailey, Mary Ann, MC, "Navigating Life's Transitions," http://www.lifetoolsforwomen.com/p/nav-lifes-transitions.htm.

[13] Ibid.

A Prayer for a Friend

This I pray for you, my friend—
That you strive to be all that you can be,
yet never become a copy of another
That you realize your own unique qualities,
and all that makes you special
That you open your eyes to the beauty
in each day
That you reach out to others less fortunate than you
That, by giving, you learn the joy of receiving…
That you let go of the sadness of the past,
yet always remember the good moments
That you learn to accept life as it is,
even with its problems and disappointments
For life is meant to be enjoyed
and, at times, endured, but never taken for granted
And I pray that you will be aware at all times
that you are one special person,
among all special persons
And do the best you can.

– Rhoda-Katie Hannan

Resources

Danskin Women's Triathlon Series,
   www.danskin.com/triathlon.html

Heart Zones USA, including the official training programs for the
   Danskin WTS, www.heartzones.com

Bailey Coaching, Mary Ann Bailey, MC, Career Coach to Mid-
   Life Professionals, www.baileycoaching.com, 206-760-0478,
   maryann@baileycoaching.com

GeezerJock magazine, www.geezerjock.com

Inside Triathlon magazine, www.insidetriathlon.com

Ironman Triathlons, www.ironman.com

Mary Meyer Life Fitness, including Open Water Swim Clinics,
   Seattle, Washington, www.marymeyerlifefitness.com/

Robin Quinn, health writer, book editor, and nutrition coach,
   www.writingandediting.biz and www.dietandlifestyle.com

Team Dream, www.teamdream.org, Derrick Q. Milligan,
   Dream Director

Team Survivor, www.teamsurvivor.org

Total Immersion Swim, www.totalimmersion.net

USA Triathlon, www.usatriathlon.org

Glossary

Because Sally Edwards, the National Spokeswoman of the Danskin Women's Triathlon Series, has left her imprint on so many triathletes, stories in this book make repeated references to what I refer to as "Sallyisms." Definitions of Sallyisms and other terms that show up in the book on a recurring basis are below. Sallyisms are marked with an asterisk.

ACSM: American College of Sports Medicine. One of the leading organizations providing certifications for fitness professionals.

body markings: In preparation for a race, it is customary to use a permanent marker to record the athlete's race number on her arms and legs. This serves to identify the athlete on the race course. At some locations, the body markings also include the athlete's age.

bricks: This is a common triathlon training term to describe a workout including two different sports. Most common is a bike ride immediately followed by a run. The term "brick" likely originated from the feeling that exists when starting to run after the bike—when your legs feel like bricks!

century ride: A 100-mile bike ride.

emotional fitness: Addressing the whole person, emotional fitness includes awareness of your own emotional state and the ability to regulate your emotional response to generate positive emotions and overcome destructive emotions.

*inner athlete: Within each and every one of us, regardless of our current level of fitness (or lack thereof), our inner athlete resides, waiting to be discovered.

Ironman: The ultimate triathlon challenge with a swim of 2.4 miles, a 112-mile bike ride, followed by a marathon (26.2-mile run). The Ironman Hawaii, held in Kona, is the "world championship" of triathlon.

*monkeys on our backs: Monkeys are the fears and self-limiting beliefs that try to prevent us from realizing our dreams. Monkeys whisper in our ears that we are too old, fat, out-of-shape—the list can go on and on—to ever be able to complete a triathlon or reach other goals in our lives.

periodization: A more advanced application of training that varies the intensity and the amount of training within a training cycle (i.e., a month) to allow the body adequate rest and recovery while improving overall fitness.

*rocks: Inevitably, on the journey to our goals, rocks appear in the form of obstacles. These obstacles can throw us off the path to achieving our goal, if we let them.

swim angels: For the swim at the Danskin triathlons, these are wonderful volunteers who line the swim route to provide support to distressed swimmers. The swim angels are in addition to the volunteer lifeguards who lend their watchful eye from boats and platforms along the swim route. Swim angels and lifeguards allow a weary or panicked swimmer to take a break, catch a breath, or regroup so she can continue to the swim finish.

Team Danskin Training (TDT): The "official training program" of the Danskin Women's Triathlon Series. Initially developed by Sally Edwards and refined by others along the way, this is an eight- or nine-week group training program. Typically, the training team works out together two times per week. Other individual workouts are assigned for the other days of the week. (Many of the stories in this book came from participants in TDT.)

Team Survivor: An organization for women who have survived cancer and now use exercise as one of their routes to recovery. At the Danskin Women's Triathlon Series, Team Survivor members start in the second wave, following the elite triathletes.

transition: The time and activities between each event of a triathlon. Transition 1 (T1) is the swim-to-bike transition. Transition 2 (T2) is the bike-to-run transition.

USAT: USA Triathlon is the sanctioning authority for more than 2,000 multisport events nationwide. USA Triathlon's 100,000-strong membership is comprised of athletes of all ages, coaches, officials, parents and fans, striving together to strengthen multisport activities.

wave: For larger triathlons, participants are started in smaller groups of typically 50-100. Most often, the "elite" or professional athletes will start in the first wave. Additional groups start at 2-5 minute intervals, typically organized by age groups.

Workout Leaders (WOLs): For each TDT group, a number of volunteers, called Workout Leaders, assist the team members and provide support as well as encouragement during training. Often WOLs were training team members the year before. They are a key component to the success of Team Danskin Training. As volunteers, their compensation is non-monetary. WOLs have extra-large hearts.

Printed in the United States
202535BV00002B/1-108/P